ADA POCKET GUIDE TO

Eating Disorders

Jessica Setnick, MS, RD, CSSD

eat right. Academy of Nutrition and Dietetics

Diana Faulhaber, Publisher
Laura Pelehach, Acquisitions and Development Manager
Elizabeth Nishiura, Production Manager

10 9 8 7 6 5 4 3 2

Library of Congress Cataloging-in-Publication Data

Setnick, Jessica.
ADA pocket guide to eating disorders / Jessica Setnick.
p. ; cm.
Pocket guide to eating disorders
Includes bibliographical references and index.
ISBN 978-0-88091-436-9
1. Eating disorders—Diet therapy—Handbooks, manuals, etc.
I. American Dietetic Association. II. Title. III. Title: Pocket guide to eating disorders.
[DNLM: 1. Eating Disorders—diet therapy—Handbooks. 2. Nutrition Assessment—Handbooks 3. Nutrition Therapy—methods—Handbooks. WM 34]
RC552.E18S48 2011
616.85'260654—dc22

2011008750

Contents

Reviewers

Roberta Anding, MS, RD, CSSD, CDE
Texas Childrens Hospital
Houston, TX

Lauren M. Carlson, MS, RD, CDN
Western Psychiatric Institute and Clinic of UPMC
Pittsburgh, PA

Diane Keddy, MS, RD, FAED
Private practice
Huntington Beach, CA

Evelyn Tribole, MS, RD
Private practice
Newport Beach, CA

Chapter 1

Eating Disorders and the Registered Dietitian

INTRODUCTION

As a food and nutrition professional, you may see eating disorders cropping up in your world at any time. Patients, coworkers, family members, and even strangers, seek out registered dietitians (RDs) for help, advice, and direction about eating disorders. Eating disorders may be your specialty treatment area, or you may specifically prefer not to treat them. In either case, you are bound to encounter them at some time in your career. They are simply too common to avoid (1).

Because nutritional rehabilitation is a cornerstone of eating disorder recovery (2), your influence as an RD can be powerful (1,3,4). Through nutrition assessment, you can identify eating disorder behaviors at their earliest stages; through nutrition education, you can raise awareness of the factors known to cause eating disorders and their signs and symptoms; through nutrition counseling, you can change the course of lives.

This pocket guide is a starting point for the RD providing medical nutrition therapy for patients with eating disorders. It includes guidelines for three steps of the Nutrition Care Process (5–7): nutrition assessment (Chapters 2 through 6), nutrition diagnosis (Chapter 7), and nutrition intervention (Chapters 8 through 11). No single book can answer all nutrition-related questions about eating disorders, and much is not known. Continuing education in this area will be necessary as new developments are made.

PREVALENCE AND DEMOGRAPHICS OF EATING DISORDERS

Rough estimates suggest that at least 13.5 million Americans meet criteria for anorexia, bulimia, or binge eating disorder (1,8–10). In a 2005 survey of 1,500 American adults, 4 out of 10 respondents said they either had or knew someone who had an eating disorder (8). As an RD, you may find that eating disorders are more common among your colleagues than in the general population (11,12). You may even have been motivated to enter the field because of your personal experiences with your own or a loved one's eating disorder (13).

Sadly, only a small fraction of individuals with eating disorders ever enter, much less complete, treatment (14). The reasons that treatment is not pursued are many, and include the following:

- Denial of the disorder and/or its severity
- Fear that recovery will involve weight gain or other undesirable consequences
- Feeling ashamed of behaviors and hiding them due to fear of embarrassment
- Cost of treatment and inadequate insurance coverage
- Failure of the medical team to consider an eating disorder diagnosis

Because many parts of our society and culture condone, encourage, and reward pathological attempts at weight control, eating disorders can avoid detection for many years—for a lifetime in some cases. A woman with anorexia is 12 times more likely to die at a young age (15) and 59 times more likely to commit suicide (16) than a woman of the same age without anorexia. Even in death, a person's eating disorder can remain unknown, as the cause of death may be listed as a more immediate event, such as heart failure or cardiac arrest.

There is no "typical" eating disorder patient in terms of demographics. Although most research subjects to date have been female, researchers now attempt to include males as well. It is dangerous and unethical to rule out an eating disorder solely on the basis of gender, socioeconomic status, weight, age, race, appearance, mental capacity, or any other single factor.

EATING DISORDERS TERMINOLOGY

"Eating disorders" is the umbrella term currently used to describe abnormal and maladaptive eating and related behaviors with psychological and biological underpinnings. In the United States, the American Psychiatric Association (APA) oversees the establishment of criteria for defining psychological conditions. These are updated and published periodically in the *Diagnostic and Statistical Manual of Mental Disorders* (DSM) (17). Because the underlying neurochemistry of eating disorders is not yet understood, the current categorization of eating disorders is based on reported symptoms and behaviors.

Eating disorders currently defined in the most recent DSM, the DSM-IV-TR, include anorexia nervosa and bulimia nervosa, with "provisional" criteria for binge eating disorder (17). For binge eating disorder and other eating disorders that do not meet the specified guidelines for anorexia or bulimia, a catch-all diagnostic category is provided. This diagnosis is "eating disorders not otherwise specified" (EDNOS). EDNOS is not an eating disorder in itself, nor should it be considered a less severe form of anorexia or bulimia. It is simply a category that can include many variations of eating disorders not yet defined. A 5th edition of the DSM, DSM-V, is expected to be published in 2013. The eating disorders section is likely to be updated with changes to the diagnostic criteria (18). Boxes 1.1 through 1.4 provide the diagnostic criteria for eating disorders as published in the DSM-IV-TR (17). The numbers in parentheses represent the associated ICD–9 codes.

Box 1.1 DSM-IV Criteria for Anorexia Nervosa (307.1)

A Refusal to maintain body weight at or above a minimally normal weight for age and height (eg, weight loss leading to maintenance of body weight less than 85% of that expected or failure to make expected weight gain during period of growth, leading to body weight less than 85% of that expected).

B Intense fear of gaining weight or becoming fat, even though underweight.

C Disturbance in the way in which one's body weight or shape is experienced, undue influence of body weight or shape on self-evaluation, or denial of the seriousness of the current low body weight.

D In postmenarcheal females, amenorrhea, ie, the absence of at least three consecutive menstrual cycles. (A woman is considered to have amenorrhea if her periods occur only following hormone, eg, estrogen, administration.)

Specify type:

Restricting type
During the current episode of anorexia nervosa, the person has not regularly engaged in binge-eating or purging behavior (ie, self-induced vomiting or the misuse of laxatives, diuretics, or enemas).

Binge eating/purging type
During the current episode of anorexia nervosa, the person has regularly engaged in a binge eating or purging behavior (ie, self-induced vomiting or the misuse of laxatives, diuretics, or enemas).

Source: Reprinted with permission from American Psychiatric Association. *Diagnostic and Statistical Manual of Mental Disorders, Fourth Edition, Text Revision.* Washington, DC: American Psychiatric Association; 2000.

Box 1.2 DSM-IV Criteria for Bulimia Nervosa (307.51)

A Recurrent episodes of binge eating, characterized by both of the following:
   (1) Eating, in a discrete period of time (eg, within any 2-hour period), an amount of food that is definitely larger than most people would eat during a similar period of time and under similar circumstances.
   (2) A sense of lack of control over eating during the episode (eg, a feeling that one cannot stop eating or control what or how much one is eating).

B Recurrent inappropriate compensatory behavior in order to prevent weight gain, such as self-induced vomiting; misuse of laxatives, diuretics, enemas, or other medications; fasting; or excessive exercise.

C The binge eating and inappropriate compensatory behaviors both occur, on average, at least twice a week for 3 months.

D Self-evaluation is unduly influenced by body shape and weight.

E The disturbance does not occur exclusively during episodes of anorexia nervosa.

Specify type:

Purging type
During the current episode of bulimia nervosa, the person has regularly engaged in self-induced vomiting or the misuse of laxatives, diuretics, or enemas.

Nonpurging type
During the current episode of bulimia nervosa, the person has used other inappropriate compensatory behaviors, such as fasting or excessive exercise, but has not regularly engaged in self-induced vomiting or the misuse of laxatives, diuretics, or enemas.

Source: Reprinted with permission from American Psychiatric Association. *Diagnostic and Statistical Manual of Mental Disorders, Fourth Edition, Text Revision.* Washington, DC: American Psychiatric Association; 2000.

Box 1.3 DSM-IV Criteria for Eating Disorder NOS (307.50)

The Eating Disorder Not Otherwise Specified category is for disorders of eating that do not meet the criteria for any specific Eating Disorder. Examples include:

1. For females, all of the criteria for Anorexia Nervosa are met except that the individual has regular menses.
2. All of the criteria for Anorexia Nervosa are met except that, despite significant weight loss, the individual's current weight is in the normal range.
3. All of the criteria for Bulimia Nervosa are met except that the binge eating and inappropriate compensatory mechanisms occur at a frequency of less than twice a week or for a duration of less than 3 months.
4. The regular use of inappropriate compensatory behavior by an individual of normal body weight after eating small amounts of food (eg, self-induced vomiting after the consumption of two cookies).
5. Repeatedly chewing and spitting out, but not swallowing, large amounts of food.
6. Binge eating disorder: recurrent episodes of binge eating in the absence of the regular use of inappropriate compensatory behaviors characteristic of Bulimia Nervosa. [See Box 1.4 for suggested research criteria.]

Source: Reprinted with permission from American Psychiatric Association. *Diagnostic and Statistical Manual of Mental Disorders, Fourth Edition, Text Revision.* Washington, DC: American Psychiatric Association; 2000.

Box 1.4 DSM-IV Research Criteria for Binge Eating Disorder

A Recurrent episodes of binge eating, characterized by both of the following:

(1) Eating, in a discrete period of time (eg, within any 2-hour period), an amount of food that is definitely larger than most people would eat during a similar period of time and under similar circumstances.

(2) A sense of lack of control over eating during the episode (eg, a feeling that one cannot stop eating or control what or how much one is eating).

B The binge eating episodes are associated with three (or more) of the following:

(1) Eating much more rapidly than normal

(2) Eating until feeling uncomfortably full

(3) Eating large amounts of food when not feeling physically hungry

(4) Eating alone because of being embarrassed by how much one is eating

(5) Feeling disgusted with oneself, depressed, or very guilty after overeating

C Marked distress regarding binge eating is present.

D The binge eating occurs, on average, at least 2 days a week for 6 months.

E The binge is not associated with the regular use of inappropriate compensatory behaviors (eg, purging, fasting, excessive exercise) and does not occur exclusively during the course of Anorexia Nervosa or Bulimia Nervosa.

Source: Reprinted with permission from American Psychiatric Association. *Diagnostic and Statistical Manual of Mental Disorders, Fourth Edition, Text Revision.* Washington, DC: American Psychiatric Association; 2000.

ETIOLOGY OF EATING DISORDERS

Binge eating, self-induced vomiting, excessive exercise, starvation, and other eating disorder behaviors are harmful and destructive, so why do they begin, and why do they persist? These questions are under investigation, but research to date has not provided any definitive answers. It seems that both biological and environmental influences contribute to the development and persistence of eating disorders (2), but the contributions of each factor and how they specifically lead to eating disorders remains unclear.

Biological Factors

Research suggests that eating disorders have genetic heritability potential (19–21). Twin studies have added pieces to the puzzle, suggesting that genetic contributions toward eating disorders may change during puberty (22), that boys with a female twin are more likely to develop an eating disorder than those with a male twin (23), and that binge eating disorder and bulimia may share genetic factors (24). Neonatal complications and maternal health during pregnancy may also influence eating disorder development (25).

It is likely that genes also play a role in the perpetuation of eating disorder behaviors once they have begun, making them more neurochemically rewarding for those with certain genes. Clues to these brain chemistry connections are provided by the frequency with which individuals with eating disorders and their family members exhibit other disorders. For example, neurochemical changes associated with eating disorder behaviors seem similar to those induced by drugs of abuse, which may mean that they soothe troubled brain chemistry in a similar manner (26,27). This may explain why individuals with eating disorders often also struggle with substance abuse disorders (28). Eating disorders can also be associated with anxiety, depression, obsessive-compulsive disorder, posttraumatic stress disorder, attention-deficit disorder, and borderline personality disorder (17). However, we do not know whether the connections are cause and effect, genetic, environmental, or a combination of these factors. Connections between eating disorders and hormonal imbalances—including polycystic ovarian syndrome, hypoglycemia, diabetes, and menstrual irregularities not specifically related to nutrition—may also be possible.

At least one type of eating disorder may be completely biological (ie, without psychological or societal influences). Pediatric autoimmune neuropsychiatric disorders associated with streptococcal infection (PANDAS) is a form of anorexia nervosa observed in pre-adolescent children who refuse to eat, leading to weight loss, within weeks of having a streptococcal infection. Little is known about PANDAS, and it is difficult to diagnose (29). Further study of PANDAS may offer greater understanding of the root causes of other types of eating disorders.

Nonbiological Factors

Current understanding of eating disorders indicates that although biology plays a role in eating disorder development, psychological, cultural, and situational stimuli also play a role. Possible contributing factors include the following:

- Voluntary and involuntary weight changes
- Traumatic stress
- Chronic stress
- Familial instability
- Physical illness or injury
- Social pressure

Weight loss, whether intentional or unintentional, may be the most immediate precursor of eating disorder development. It is well understood that restriction of energy intake can lead to biochemical and psychological changes that resemble eating disorders. What is not understood is why some energy-restricted individuals develop eating disorders, whereas others do not. One theory is that the social effects of weight changes can be dramatically negative or positive when a culture overvalues a slender body shape and size. Therefore, regardless of an individual's original intention to lose or gain weight, criticism or praise for doing so may trigger an eating disorder if the individual is biologically susceptible.

Weight changes that lead to eating disorders are often preceded by one or more traumatic events (30,31). The biochemical effects of starvation might be more strongly felt by individuals in emotional distress. In these cases, the desire for weight loss may derive from an attempt to modulate stressful feelings—what is often described as an effort to regain a sense of "control" (2). Because eating disorder behaviors can create a temporary feeling of well-being (by changing brain chemistry), they can create a positive feedback loop to perpetuate the behaviors, even beyond the point where they become harmful or life threatening.

THE RD'S ROLE

As an RD, you must perform within the ethical scope of practice defined by your registration and licensure. Currently, no officially sanctioned guidelines specifically define the RD's role in eating disorders treatment, although these are in development. Your facility may provide you with a job description, but it is likely that the actual expectations and demands of your role will differ from the specifications detailed there, especially if the job description is for the general role of RD rather than specific to eating disorders treatment. Box 1.5 lists some of the functions an RD may play in the treatment of eating disorders.

Box 1.5 Role of the Registered Dietitian in the Treatment of Eating Disorders

- Evaluate the patient's current eating patterns and develop a plan for improvement.
- Share with other team members any nutrition information that may affect the patient's physical and mental health or medication needs.
- Construct a healthy eating pattern individualized to each patient to address current nutrition concerns and physical needs.
- Help the patient establish this healthy eating pattern.
- Challenge food myths, misconceptions, and harmful beliefs.
- Explain the role of proper nutrition and food in physical and mental health.
- Identify disordered eating behaviors that interfere with proper nutrition.
- Help resolve disordered thoughts and feelings around food, eating, and body size.
- Refer information discovered about underlying stress issues to the mental health therapist.
- When appropriate, offer active learning activities, such as cooking, therapeutic meals, or grocery shopping, to help teach new behaviors and acceptance of food-related tasks and environments. Model appropriate eating at therapeutic meals.
- Communicate frequently with other members of the interdisciplinary treatment team regarding nutrition interventions and the patient's health status.
- Teach group nutrition classes and/or lead group nutrition discussions.
- Educate parents and caregivers regarding eating disorders and/or nutrition.
- Avoid inserting personal eating preferences or bias into nutrition education.

Because the role of the RD in the treatment of eating disorders may be interpreted differently by your supervisor, other professionals you work with, and even other RDs, you may at times experience concern that you are stepping outside of the RD's appropriate scope of practice. Alternatively, you may think that your official job responsibilities are too limiting. In these situations, consult a supervisor, mentor, colleague, or other adviser. The person who hired you may not necessarily be familiar with the role of the RD, or the part the RD plays on the eating disorders treatment team. With patience, you can help educate yourself and those you work with about your role.

ARE YOU READY?

Every RD has something to offer to a patient with an eating disorder. The primary requirement is an interest in the field and willingness to learn. Even your nonjudgmental response to a patient's description of eating disorder behaviors can be in its own small way a meaningful intervention (32). At the same time, eating disorders care is a specialty area that requires additional training (such as continuing education and on-the-job training) beyond what is provided in school and traditional dietetics training programs (17).

If you find yourself doubting your abilities or "taking your work home with you," know that these are common reactions to working with individuals with eating disorders, not signs that you are inadequate. Even the most experienced clinicians recognize that working with individuals in various stages of illness and recovery from eating disorders offers daily challenges that are not related to "knowing enough" or "doing enough." The fact that you are reading this book shows that you are attempting to enlarge your knowledge base and your competence level. Further education and confidence-building can be found at continuing education seminars and conferences targeted toward RDs and/or mental health professionals; in professional support and networking groups; and through case conferences with your treatment team. Do not be afraid to admit that you find a particular situation or patient stressful, as this is normal, and keeping these feelings inside can lead to anxiety, unprofessional behavior, and "burnout." If your contact with other, more experienced professionals at your workplace is limited, consider seeking mentoring or case consultation (also called "professional supervision") from a more experienced RD or mental health professional, either in person or by phone.

If you realize that you are not interested in the field, you do not feel sympathetic toward individuals with eating disorders, or you get easily frustrated with slow or little progress, you may choose not to seek out this patient population. However, you may still occasionally encounter a patient with an eating disorder. In these instances, speak with your supervisor for guidance, refer the patient to a different RD, and ensure that you have moral support to help you cope with what can be a stressful situation.

Finally, if you realize that you are struggling with your own eating issues, or if you recognize that your work is triggering unhealthy thoughts or behaviors, know that these concerns do not disqualify you from working as an RD. You need to seek help, and you may choose not to work with this patient population for a period of time. It is not necessary to be a "perfect" eater to help others. However, you must be aware of your own thoughts, stressors, and behaviors, and be actively working in recovery. This ensures that you are able to meet a patient's needs without disregarding your own, and vice versa. A meeting with an experienced mental health professional is a good place to start. During this time, you should not discuss your eating disorder or recovery with your patients, but you can silently be a role model and show that difficulties can be overcome.

REFERENCES

1. Bruce B, Wilfley D. Binge eating among the overweight population: a serious and prevalent problem. *J Am Diet Assoc.* 1996;96:58–61.
2. Yager J, Devlin MJ, Halmi KA, Herzog DB, Mitchell JE, Powers P, Zerbe KJ. *Practice Guideline for the Treatment of Patients with Eating Disorders.* 3rd ed. Arlington, VA: American Psychiatric Association; 2006.
3. Bruce B, Agras WS. Binge eating in females: a population-based investigation. *Int J Eat Disorder.* 1992;12:365–373.
4. American Dietetic Association. Position of the American Dietetic Association: Nutrition intervention in the treatment of anorexia nervosa, bulimia nervosa, and other eating disorders. *J Am Diet Assoc.*; 2006;106:2073–2082.
5. Writing Group of the Nutrition Care Process/Standardized Language Committee. Nutrition Care Process and Model part I: the 2008 update. *J Am Diet Assoc.* 2008;108:1113–1117.
6. Writing Group of the Nutrition Care Process/Standardized Language Committee. Nutrition Care Process and Model part II: Using the International Dietetics and Nutrition Terminology to document the Nutrition Care Process. *J Am Diet Assoc.* 2008;108:1287–1293.
7. *International Dietetics & Nutrition Terminology (IDNT) Reference Manual: Standardized Language for the Nutrition Care Process.* 3rd ed. Chicago, IL: American Dietetic Association; 2011.
8. National Eating Disorders Association. American Public Opinion on Eating Disorders. http://www.nationaleatingdisorders.org/uploads/file/Statistics%20%20Updated%20Feb%2010,%202008%20B.pdf. Accessed August 10, 2010.
9. Marcus MD, Wing RR. Binge eating among the obese. *Ann Behav Med.* 1987;9:23.

10. Spitzer RL, Devlin M, Walsh BT, Hasin D, Wing R, Marcus M, Stunkard AJ, Wadden T, Yanovski S, Agras WS, Mitchell J, Nonas C. Binge eating disorder: a multisite trial for the diagnostic criteria. *Int J Eat Disorder*. 1993;11:191–203.
11. Kinzl JA, Traweger CM, Trefalt E, Mangweth B, Biebl W. Dietitians: are they a risk group for eating disorders? *Eur Eat Disord Rev*. 1999;7:62–67.
12. Worobey J, Schoenfeld D. Eating disordered behavior in dietetics students and students in other majors. *J Am Diet Assoc*. 1999;99:1100–1102.
13. Hughes R, Desbrow B. Aspiring dietitians study: a pre-enrollment study of students' motivations, awareness, and expectations relating to careers in nutrition and dietetics. *Nutr Diet*. 2005;62:106–109.
14. Striegel-Moore RH, Leslie D, Petrill SA, Garvin V, Rosenheck RA. One year use and cost of inpatient and outpatient services among female and male patients with an eating disorder: evidence from a national database of insurance claims. *Int J Eat Disord*. 2000;27:381–389.
15. Sullivan PF. Mortality in anorexia nervosa. *Am J Psychiatry*.1995;152:1073–1074.
16. Keel PK, Dorer DJ, Eddy KT, Franko D, Charatan DL, Herzog DB. Predictors of mortality in eating disorders. *Arch Gen Psychiatry*. 2003;60:179–183.
17. American Psychiatric Association. *The Diagnostic and Statistical Manual of Mental Disorders*. 4th ed, text revision. Arlington, VA: American Psychiatric Association; 2000.
18. Walsh BT. *Report of the DSM-V Eating Disorders Work Group*. August 2008. http://www.psych.org/MainMenu/Research/DSMIV/DSMV/DSMRevisionActivities/DSMVWorkGroupReports/EatingDisordersWorkGroupReport.aspx. Accessed August 10, 2010.
19. Lilenfeld LR, Kaye WH, Greeno CG, Merikangas KR, Plotnicov L, Pollice C, Rao R, Strober M, Bulik CM, Nagy L. A controlled family study of anorexia nervosa and bulimia nervosa. *Arch Gen Psychiatry*. 1998;55:603–610.
20. Strober M, Lampert C, Morrell W, Burroughs J, Jacob C. A controlled family study of anorexia nervosa: evidence of familial aggregation and lack of shared transmission with affective disorders. *Int J Eat Disorder*. 1990;9:239–253

21. Grice DA, Halmi KA, Fichter MM, Strober M, Woodside DB, Treasure JT, Kaplan AS, Magistretti PJ, Goldman D, Bulik CM, Kaye WH, Berrettini WH. Evidence for a susceptibility gene for anorexia nervosa on chromosome 1. *Am J Hum Genet.* 2002;70:787–792.
22. Klump KL, Burt SA, McGue M, Iacono WG. Changes in genetic and environmental influences on disordered eating across adolescence: a longitudinal twin study. *Arch Gen Psychiatry.* 2007;64:1409–1415.
23. Procopio M, Marriott P. Intrauterine hormonal environment and risk of developing anorexia nervosa. *Arch Gen Psychiatry.* 2007;64:1402–1407.
24. Wade TD, Bulik CM, Sullivan PF, Neale MC, Kendler KS. The relation between risk factors for binge eating and bulimia nervosa: a population-based female twin study. *Health Psychol.* 2000;19:115–123.
25. Favaro A, Tenconi E, Santonastaso P. Perinatal factors and the risk of developing anorexia nervosa and bulimia nervosa. *Arch Gen Psychiatry.* 2006;63:82–88.
26. Wang G, Volkow ND, Thanos PK, Fowler JS. Similarity between obesity and drug addiction as assessed by neurofunctional imaging: a concept review. *J Addict Dis.* 2004;23:39–53.
27. Kalra SP, Kalra PS. Overlapping and interactive pathways regulation appetite and craving. *J Addict Dis.* 2004;23:5–21.
28. Helfman BL, Dennis AB. Understanding the complex relationship between eating disorders and substance use disorders. *Renfrew Perspect.* 2010;(Winter):2–4.
29. Vincenzi B, O'Toole J, Lask B. PANDAS and anorexia nervosa—a spotters' guide: suggestions for medical assessment. *Eur Eat Disord Rev.* 2010;18:116–123.
30. Berg FM. *Women Afraid to Eat: Breaking Free in Today's Weight-Obsessed World.* Hettinger, MD: Healthy Weight Network; 2000.
31. Vredrvelt P, Newman D, Beverly H, Minirth F. *The Thin Disguise: Understanding and Overcoming Anorexia and Bulimia.* Nashville, TN: Thomas Nelson; 1992.
32. Kellogg M. *Counseling Tips for Nutrition Therapists: Practice Workbook.* Vol 1. Philadelphia, PA: Kg Press; 2006.

Chapter 2

Nutrition Assessment Overview

INTRODUCTION

The Nutrition Care Process begins with nutrition assessment (1–3). Registered dietitians (RDs) gather the nutrition assessment data from the person or facility making the referral, the patient's medical records, and the patient and family. Nutrition assessment is an ongoing process that involves not only initial data collection, but also reassessment and analysis of client data and needs.

INPATIENT VS OUTPATIENT SETTINGS

Depending on the setting in which you work as an RD, you will encounter patients with eating disorders in varying stages of illness, recovery, and motivation to change. Accordingly, your role may change as a patient progresses through the continuum of care.

Inpatient

In a treatment center or hospital, a thorough nutrition assessment helps determine the care plan and the goals set by the treatment team. It should be performed as soon as is reasonable after admission.

Medically unstable patients may require nutrition support on an emergency basis before a thorough nutrition assessment can be performed, and patients who are extremely malnourished, uncooperative, or hostile (such as those who are hospitalized against their will) may need time to adjust before meeting productively with you. In these cases, a preliminary nutrition assessment should be drafted from medical records and reports from family members and other care providers.

Outpatient

In an outpatient setting, the information available prior to the nutrition assessment may be more limited than in an inpatient setting. Even when patients are accompanied by a significant other, family member(s), or caregiver(s), more voices do not always provide more useful information. Other parties may not be fully aware of the patient's eating disorder behaviors, and there may be differences of opinion regarding severity, frequency, and duration of symptoms. In these cases, the nutrition assessment may take place over the course of several meetings. Patients who have been concealing their behaviors may not be used to honest disclosure and may minimize or deny their eating disorder out of fear of punishment or other negative consequences. They may need a few sessions with you before determining that you are dependable and worth trusting. See Box 2.1 for tips on establishing trust (4–6).

Box 2.1 Establishing Trust with Patients

- Ask patients about their past experiences with treatment and treatment providers.
- Allow patients to express what they did and did not like about past providers, and listen to what they say.
- Resist the urge to agree with any derogatory remarks a patient makes about past caregivers or treatment programs. Keep in mind that effective eating disorder treatment can be difficult, painful, and even involuntary; therefore, a patient may harbor negative memories of what was excellent treatment. At the same time, resist the urge to defend past caregivers or treatment programs, even if you feel the criticism is unjust. However, if you are concerned that a patient's report of past treatment indicates a violation of law or ethical conduct, speak with your supervisor, who can follow your facility's procedures for this type of situation.
- Be extra-sensitive if your initial nutrition assessment is the first time a patient has ever spoken about his or her eating disorder, or spoken about it to a professional. These situations carry additional significance, as the patient's experience of this encounter with you has the potential to influence his or her willingness to pursue recovery in general. In these cases, your nonjudgmental acceptance of the patient's experience, together with your expressions of compassion and hope are important facets of building trust (4–6).
- Do not delay in referring patients for additional treatment that you feel is needed (see Chapter 11 for more information about coordination of care). If a patient asks you not to speak with other treatment providers, explain that this is a requirement of working with you. Do not allow a patient's fears of disclosure to hamper the care you provide. Do not collude with a patient in keeping an eating disorder secret from other care providers. Seek advice from a supervisor or trusted colleague if a patient in this situation refuses additional care, especially medical attention.
- Allow enough time for a thorough evaluation, or plan a brief introduction followed by a lengthier session. Patients may

(continues next page)

Box 2.1 Establishing Trust with Patients (continued)

enter the evaluation with many psychological defenses (see Chapter 10) and will require a calm environment in order to "let down their guard" and provide you with necessary information.

- Let the patient know what your plan of action will be once you leave the session—eg, "After I leave, I'm going to send a note to the kitchen about your meal plan and call your counselor to open the lines of communication." This allows the patient to see that you are acting in a transparent manner and do not intend to keep secrets from him/her.
- Follow through on any commitments you make to a patient during your evaluation, such as "I will call your doctor and let him/her know you have a question"; "I will check with the kitchen about making that change to your menu"; and so on. This helps reinforce that you are a trustworthy person and encourages disclosure.

FAMILY PARTICIPATION

If family members are in attendance at the nutrition assessment, it is usually appropriate to request at least a few minutes alone with the patient. Check your facility's protocol and request the permission of the patient (and the patient's caregivers if the patient is a minor).

Some patients may resist talking with you alone, preferring the company of a spouse, family member, or other support person. In these cases, speak directly to the patient during the nutrition assessment, but allow the presence of the requested companion. Observe whether a patient responds differently to questions when accompanied by family members compared with when he or she is alone with you. If the responses are vastly different, you may need to involve other members of the treatment team (see Box 2.2).

Box 2.2 What to Do When Patient Responses Vary in the Presence of Family

If a patient responds one way when you talk one-on-one but gives other, notably different answers in the presence of family, here are some approaches to consider:

- When alone with the patient, ask, "Are there things that you don't like to talk about when your family/family member is in the room?" Assure the patient that you have no reason to reveal this information to other members of the family, and that you are grateful that the patient is willing to share this personal information with you because it contributes to your efforts to help. Let other treatment team members know of this interaction.
- Take care to stay within the registered dietitian's scope of practice. If you discover, for example, that a patient is concealing an eating behavior from her husband, it is not your responsibility to inform the husband or to convince the patient to tell her husband. Instead, tell the patient that you think the act of concealment is significant, and that you would like the patient to discuss this topic with her counselor. You can then alert the counselor of the conversation and your recommendation. In this way you have helped the patient address an important issue without exceeding your scope of practice as a registered dietitian.
- If you learn that in addition to concealing information from family members, a patient is concealing information from another member of the treatment team (eg, he has not shared his excessive alcohol intake with his physician), state without judgment that this is important information and ask the patient if he would prefer that you convey the information, or if he would prefer to do so. Do not accept an option in which the information continues to be concealed.
- If a patient reveals to you in confidence that he or she is engaging in dangerous behavior, whether nutrition-related or not, contact another member of the treatment team to request assistance in determining a course of action. Tell the patient that you are doing so, or place a call in the presence of the patient, but do not allow the patient to convince you to conceal the dangerous behavior.

INTERVIEWING PATIENTS

During the initial nutrition assessment, use verbal and nonverbal cues from the patient to guide the meeting to provide you with the information you need. Limit in-depth nutrition education or lengthy explanations in this first meeting, unless specifically requested by the patient, as your goal is to gather information that will help you set priorities for nutrition intervention.

Outgoing Patients

Patients who are very talkative may benefit from redirection ("That would be a great topic for your counseling session"). Try to guide them toward the information you need to gather by bridging from their preferred topic to yours ("I'm interested in hearing more about how that affects your eating").

Withdrawn Patients

Patients who are withdrawn may be comforted by reassurances that eating is a very personal topic and you appreciate their willingness to speak with you. Reiterate your confidentiality policy and ask if the patient is worrying about anything regarding this meeting, in which case you would be happy to try to reassure them.

Appropriate Terminology and Questions

Unless the patient is a medical professional, use general terminology during the nutrition assessment rather than technical or eating disorder–specific language. (For example, ask, "Do you ever feel guilty after you eat?" rather than "Do you purge?") (6). This approach helps you ask follow-up questions about the patient's specific behaviors ("What do you do when you feel that way?" "Do you do it every time that you eat, or only in certain situations?"). The use of general terminology and individualized questions also helps you avoid suggesting new eating disorder behaviors.

Suggested sample questions are listed in Boxes 2.3 and 2.4 (6). Pick and choose the questions that seem appropriate based on your preliminary knowledge of the patient's situation, and adapt as you continue.

Box 2.3 Food and Eating-Related Nutrition Assessment Questions

- Can you bring me up to date on what brought you here?
  - If the patient denies having an eating disorder or states, "I'm only here because [someone else] thinks I have a problem," ask, "What is your understanding of why [that person] wanted you to be here?"
- Can you describe your eating on a typical day?
  - Ask about the timing and content of meals/snacks.
  - Ask about the timing and quantities of noncaloric and nonnutritional foods and beverages, such as condiments, water, artificial sweeteners, coffee, chewing gum, alcohol, "energy" drinks, and so on. Note any abnormal intake.
  - Follow up if patient specifies "on a good day" or "on a bad day." Ask what, in their opinion, makes their eating "good" or "bad" and how often each type of day occurs.
- Are you allergic to any foods? Are there other foods that you don't eat? What are the reasons you don't eat those foods?
- Do you ever worry that you'll lose control around food, and eat much more than you wanted to? Is this just a worry, or does it sometimes happen?
- Can you give me an example of what you might eat that feels like "way too much"? How often does this happen?
- Which foods are your "weaknesses"? Do you try to avoid them? What happens when you are around them?
- Do you ever eat in secret? Can you describe why you feel like you need to hide?
- Do you get up in the middle of the night to eat? Are you awake or asleep when this happens?
- Do you ever wake up to find evidence of eating that surprises you?
- Do you ever have trouble keeping your food down?

(continues next page)

Box 2.3 Food and Eating-Related Nutrition Assessment Questions (continued)

- Do you ever feel guilty after you eat? Do you ever do anything about it?
- Do you ever feel like you have to "get rid of" your food?
- Is there anything special you need to do with your food?
  - Ask this as an open-ended question.
  - Possible responses from the patient might include cutting food into many tiny pieces; reheating food during a meal; drawing out a meal for a certain length of time; eating only with certain dishware or flatware; measuring or weighing portions before eating; eating only a certain number of items at a time (eg, everything in threes); and other food "rituals."
- Is there anything else you think is related to your eating that I haven't thought to ask?

Source: Adapted with permission Setnick J. *The Eating Disorders Clinical Pocket Guide: Quick Reference for Healthcare Providers*. Dallas, TX: Snack Time Press; 2005.

Box 2.4 Physical Activity-Related Nutrition Assessment Questions

- How often do you exercise?
- For how long?
- What types of activities/exercises do you do?
- Can you miss a day of exercise?
- Is your eating different on a day you exercise compared with a day you don't exercise?
- Is there anything specific that you do every time you exercise? (ie, exercise rituals)
- Have any other health providers made recommendations about the amount or type of activities you should do? Have they given you any restrictions or limits on activities?
- Do you ever exercise even though you're not supposed to?

Source: Adapted with permission from Setnick J. *The Eating Disorders Clinical Pocket Guide: Quick Reference for Healthcare Providers*. Dallas, TX: Snack Time Press; 2005.

Some answers will require follow-up questions. Keep in mind that your initial goal is not to gather every possible fact about this patient, but rather to obtain baseline information that you can use to make recommendations and build rapport and trust. If treatment continues, you will meet with the patient many more times and continue to gather (and provide) information during each session.

ORGANIZING THE WRITTEN NUTRITION ASSESSMENT

Once you have completed your interview with the patient and family members, reviewed any anthropometric data and/or written documentation you have obtained, and gathered any information available from the patient's medical record, you will document your findings and recommendations. Your written assessment of an eating disorder patient will likely touch on all five categories of the Nutrition Care Process nutrition assessment data:

- Food/nutrition-related history (Chapter 3)
- Anthropometric measurements (Chapter 4)
- Biochemical data, medical tests, and procedures (Chapter 4)
- Nutrition-focused physical findings (Chapter 5)
- Client history, including social and medical history (Chapter 6)

Once your assessment is complete, you will have a basis to determine your patient's nutrition diagnosis (see Chapter 7).

REFERENCES

1. Writing Group of the Nutrition Care Process/Standardized Language Committee. Nutrition Care Process and Model part I: the 2008 update. *J Am Diet Assoc.* 2008;108:1113–1117.
2. Writing Group of the Nutrition Care Process/Standardized Language Committee. Nutrition Care Process and Model part II: Using the International Dietetics and Nutrition Terminology to document the Nutrition Care Process. *J Am Diet Assoc.* 2008;108:1287–1293.
3. *International Dietetics & Nutrition Terminology (IDNT) Reference Manual: Standardized Language for the Nutrition Care Process.* 3rd ed. Chicago, IL: American Dietetic Association; 2011.
4. Kellogg M. *Counseling Tips for Nutrition Therapists: Practice Workbook.* Vol 2. Philadelphia, PA: Kg Press; 2009.
5. Yager J, Devlin MJ, Halmi KA, Herzog DB, Mitchell JE, Powers P, Zerbe KJ. *Practice Guideline for the Treatment of Patients with Eating Disorders.* 3rd ed. Arlington, VA: American Psychiatric Association; 2006.
6. Setnick J. *The Eating Disorders Clinical Pocket Guide: Quick Reference for Healthcare Providers.* Dallas, TX: Snack Time Press; 2005.

Chapter 3

Nutrition Assessment of Food and Nutrition-Related History

INTRODUCTION

This chapter addresses nutrition assessment topics that the International Dietetics and Nutrition Terminology (IDNT) categorizes in the domain of Food and Nutrition-related History (1). Topics include food and nutrient intake; diet experience; medication and supplement use; behavior; beliefs and attitudes; food and nutrition-related knowledge; food availability; and physical activity.

FOOD AND NUTRIENT INTAKE

Clearly, a key to the nutrition assessment of a patient with a diagnosed or suspected eating disorder is the assessment of what he or she eats and drinks. In the hospital setting, note intake since admission as well as usual (reported) intake prior to hospitalization. In the outpatient setting, "usual" intake may vary greatly from day to day, or it can be rigidly routine. In some cases, a patient may be an excellent historian, in others, accurate information about intake can be notoriously difficult to obtain. (See Box 3.1 for information on the use of food diaries in the nutrition assessment of patients with eating disorders.) The following sections identify some of the key aspects of intake to assess and note their relationship to eating disorders. These findings may then lead to nutrition diagnoses (Chapter 7) and nutrition interventions (Chapters 8 through 11).

Box 3.1 Food Diaries and Nutrition Assessment

A food diary can be a useful tool for recording food intake in situ, rather than expecting a patient to remember everything that was ingested. Inpatient food diaries are often simple calorie counts or percentages of food eaten, and are usually completed by nursing staff. You may ask that patients keep an additional log of other information you or other members of the treatment team would like to gather. This may include reasons that a patient did not complete a meal or eat certain foods; feelings or thoughts before and/or after eating; temptations to purge, restrict or exercise; and so on.

Patients in the outpatient setting may keep track of any or all of those items, plus hunger and/or fullness cues; environmental influences on eating; time and/or duration of meals; measurements of portion sizes; and/or other details that you believe will provide useful information.

For some patients, completing a food diary is more important as an accountability tool ("I'd better eat my meal because my dietitian will see my food diary") than as a source of information. These patients may simply prefer a check-off sheet that indicates whether or not they completed a meal, or a sign-off sheet that a family member initials to indicate that a meal was completed, rather than a food diary per se.

You may encounter patients who refuse to keep a food diary, who believe that a food diary will worsen obsessive thoughts about food, or who have been traumatized by keeping a food diary in a punitive manner. Explain to such patients why you are asking for a food diary (you would like to observe patterns of eating and behavior that will allow you to create a treatment plan), and address any reservations the patient has (you will not be grading the food diary nor chastising the patient for eating that differs from recommendations). These reassurances may allow the patient to reconsider. Offer alternatives,

(continues next page)

Box 3.1 Food Diaries and Nutrition Assessment (continued)

such as e-mailing a food record at the end of each day (if this is acceptable to you) so that there is no document that could be found by roommates or family members, or a check-off list as mentioned previously.

In situations where a patient will under no circumstances keep a food diary or simply expresses that he or she "doesn't want to," two options remain—a family member records the patient's intake (with or without the patient's permission), or the patient provides a verbal recall. Some patients, upon realizing how difficult it is to remember everything they ate and/or that you really are not going to judge their intake, will agree to keep a food diary after all. Others will continue to provide information verbally.

ENERGY INTAKE

The nutrition assessment of energy intake should evaluate the "amount of energy intake from all sources, eg, food, beverages, supplements, and via enteral and parenteral routes" (1).

Inadequate energy intake is inherent in the diagnosis of anorexia nervosa. The energy intake of patients who engage in binge/fast cycles may also be inadequate. Patients diagnosed with an eating disorder not otherwise specified (EDNOS) because they do not meet weight criteria for anorexia may consume inadequate calories in an effort to lose weight or to compensate after bingeing (2). It is important not to dismiss the possibility of inadequate energy intake simply because an individual presents with a normal or above-normal weight.

FLUID INTAKE

Assess the "amount and type of fluid/beverage intake consumed orally" (1). Patients may avoid or limit fluid intake to reduce body weight. Fluid restriction is common among the following:

- Athletes required to "weigh in"
- Individuals who want to lose weight rapidly
- Those who fear that fluids cause "bloating"
- Those who wish to avoid the feeling of anything in the stomach

FOOD INTAKE

For each patient, the registered dietitian (RD) should assess the "amount, type, and pattern of food consumed and quality of diet" (1). Indicators include the amount of food eaten from the various food groups, percent of total meal eaten, types of food/meals consumed, the number of meals and snacks eaten daily, and food variety. Note that eating patterns and food intake may vary considerably from day to day.

Types of Food/Meals

Individuals attempting to reduce their intake of calories and unwanted or feared nutrients may choose processed foods (such as "energy" bars, "sport" drinks, and "energy" drinks) over fresh or homemade foods. They may perceive the processed foods to be more portion-controlled and the nutrition information more standardized. Depending on the individually preferred foods, intake of supplemental vitamins and minerals from these foods may be excessive.

If patients primarily eat convenience foods, pre-prepared meals, and foods prepared away from home, their intake of sodium may be excessive and their intake of healthful nutrients may be inadequate.

Some patients with eating disorders limit themselves to "filler" foods—bulky, nutrient-poor foods such as rice cakes and bran cereal—that will provide a physical feeling of fullness with few calories. This type of eating can result in excessive fiber intake, constipation, inadequate nutrient intake, and limited absorption of some micronutrients.

See Box 3.2 for information on food faddism and pica.

Box 3.2 Food Faddism and Pica

Dangers of food faddism and pica range from poor nutrition to intestinal blockage. Assess whether the patient ingests either of the following:

- Nonfood substances intended to induce feelings of fullness without calories (such as fiber tablets, sugar-free chewing gum, or cotton balls)
- Excessive quantities of foods reputed to cause weight loss (such as grapefruit or celery)

This information should be provided to the medical professional along with any reports of gastrointestinal distress.

Note that individuals reporting excessive chewing of gum, writing utensils, drinking straws, fingernails, ice, or crunchy foods should be referred for an evaluation by a mental health professional as they may indicate the presence of high anxiety. A craving for ice and excessive chewing of ice may be a symptom of iron-deficiency anemia and should be evaluated by a medical professional.

Food Variety (Present/Absent)

Assess any restrictions the patient makes when choosing foods or food groups. In the assessment, consider psychological and physical factors that may contribute to the restriction of food choices. (See Box 3.3; see also "Avoidance Behavior," later in this chapter.)

Box 3.3 Intake on "Good" and "Bad" Days

Many patients with eating disorders will describe drastically varying eating patterns, often described as "good days" and "bad days." It is helpful to find out what constitutes the difference in intake; why this is perceived as "good/healthy/acceptable" or "bad/unhealthy/unacceptable"; and what triggers each type of day to occur.

Some food restrictions may be related to gastrointestinal (GI) distress, which the patient may attribute to food intolerance, but which may also be caused by fasting, bingeing, purging, and any combination of these behaviors. The symptoms may be due to the eating disorder, or the eating disorder may have developed as an individual eliminated different foods in an attempt to find the source of the GI problem.

Reports of food sensitivities and allergies should be assessed and taken into account during nutritional restoration, with the caveat that some foods may not require restriction once normal digestive function has been restored. Other reasons individuals with eating disorders may avoid certain foods include the following:

- Individuals with hemorrhoids or other conditions that make elimination painful may prefer not to eat at all.
- Athletes may avoid eating before competition, so they will not need to empty their bladder or bowels during the event.
- Patients may have mistaken beliefs that individual foods are responsible for weight gain.
- Patients may fear that eating even a small amount of a food will trigger a binge.

Recent Changes in Food Intake

Changes in food intake may not be recognized as the signals of emotional distress that they often are. When a patient suddenly changes his or her eating pattern or begins to avoid foods, it is essential to investigate what caused or instigated the change.

Something seemingly innocuous—a comment from a friend, an unexceptional doctor's appointment, a television commercial—can trigger a change in eating in a susceptible individual. If the trigger is identified early enough, an eating disorder may possibly be averted, and the root of the issue—whether anxiety, hurt feelings, misinformation, or some other factor—can be addressed.

ENTERAL AND PARENTERAL INTAKE

A patient who is emaciated from starvation or unable to keep food down may require assistance and/or nutrition support in order to obtain adequate nutrition. For more information on enteral and parenteral nutrition, see Chapter 8.

MACRONUTRIENT INTAKE

In the assessment of the patient's macronutrient intake, consider "fat and cholesterol, protein, carbohydrate, and fiber intake from all sources, including food, beverages, supplements, and via enteral and parenteral nutrition" (1).

Fats

Fat is arguably the nutrient most commonly restricted by individuals with eating disorders. Patients may avoid dietary fat because they have read that it contains more calories per gram than other nutrients, because they believe that foods containing fat are "fattening," and/or because of the semantic association between dietary "fat," body "fat," and being "fat." Consequences of inadequate fat intake may include limited food variety and poor absorption of fat-soluble nutrients (3).

Adequate essential fatty acid intake is necessary for proper brain function and eating disorder recovery. Chronic fatty acid deficiency can also affect liver function. Increased liver enzymes due to fatty acid deficiency should be monitored by a physician and often decrease over time as nutrition is restored.

Protein

Patients with eating disorders may consume excessive amounts of protein in a misguided attempt to protect muscle mass during weight loss. This is especially common in men and athletes of both genders with eating disorders. Conversely, some girls and women with eating disorders avoid eating food sources of protein because they mistakenly believe that it will cause their muscles to grow and they wish to avoid looking "muscular" or "bulky."

Carbohydrate

Patients may not accurately understand which foods contain carbohydrate, as the general label "carbs" has been popularly applied to a variety of foods from whole grains to potatoes to fruit. If your patient reports limiting "carbs," clarify which foods he or she includes in this category.

VITAMIN AND MINERAL INTAKE

Assess micronutrient intake from all sources—food, beverages, supplements, and via enteral and parenteral routes (1).

Eating disorders, including overeating disorders, can result in nutritional deficiencies related to food restrictions and rituals. Some individuals with eating disorders refuse to take a multivitamin/mineral or other supplement to replenish nutrient stores, because they believe that supplements contain calories or will increase appetite.

On the other hand, patients who are aware that their dietary intake is inadequate may ingest excessive nutrients by self-prescribing vitamin and/or mineral supplements in a misguided attempt to maintain health (3).

See Chapter 8 for additional information about micronutrient deficiencies.

BIOACTIVE SUBSTANCES INTAKE

Alcohol

Assess the amount and pattern of alcohol consumption (1). Alcohol use is linked to disordered eating, even in the absence of alcohol dependence (alcoholism) (4,5). Individuals who consume alcohol may skip meals or induce vomiting to "save calories" for drinking ("drinkorexia").

Caffeine and Other Stimulants

Assess the amount of caffeine from all sources (food, beverages, supplements, medications, and via enteral and parenteral routes) (1). Drinking coffee (or ingesting instant coffee crystals or coffee beans), tea, caffeinated carbonated beverages and "energy" drinks can result in an excessive intake of caffeine and other stimulants (4,6). See Appendix B for data on the levels of caffeine in selected foods, beverages, supplements, and medications.

Some patients are unaware of the role that caffeine and other stimulants play in their eating disorder. Other patients may consciously use stimulants for one or more of the following reasons:

- To depress or mask appetite
- To maintain energy levels in the face of inadequate calorie intake
- To propel excessive exercise
- To self-medicate for attention deficit disorder, anxiety, or chronic fatigue (if this is suspected, a physician evaluation should be recommended)
- To combat cold-intolerance by drinking hot (and caffeinated) beverages

Excessive intake of caffeine can induce insomnia, anxiety, and/or caffeine intoxication (see Box 3.4) (4). Caffeine dependence may require a weaning process to prevent physical symptoms of withdrawal (most notably severe headache) (4).

Box 3.4 Symptoms of Caffeine Intoxication

- Gastrointestinal disturbance
- Rambling thoughts/speech
- Agitation
- Muscle twitching

Source: Data are from reference 4.

MEDICATION AND HERBAL SUPPLEMENTS

In the assessment of a patient's use of medications and supplements, consider "prescription and over-the counter medications, including herbal preparations and complementary medicine products that may impact nutritional status" (1). Eating disorder patients can become physiologically and/or psychologically dependent on medications and even dietary supplements.

Patients should be discouraged from using supplements called "fat-blockers" or "carb-blockers" as well as any kind of diet pill—even if they are not effective, these products still encourage the eating disorder mentality and can exacerbate GI disturbances. Whether self-prescribed or recommended by a friend or pseudo-health professional, all such substances should be evaluated by the physician.

See Box 3.5 for selected types of medications that may exacerbate eating disorder symptoms (7,8). Refer to Chapter 8 for information on the nutrition-related effects of psychoactive medications.

Box 3.5 Selected Medications Relevant to Nutrition Assessment of Eating Disorders[a]

- **Medications associated with weight loss, anorexia, or increased energy expenditure**: Any medication that leads to weight loss, whether as its main purpose or as a side effect, has the potential to trigger an eating disorder in a susceptible individual. If the medication is used temporarily, patients may restrict eating after its use is discontinued because they fear weight gain.
- **Lipid-lowering medications**: Some patients generally avoid medications and prefer to attempt lifestyle interventions exclusively. When patients have elevated serum lipid levels, their physicians may offer a timeline, such as 6 weeks or 3 months, to improve the lipid levels via "diet and exercise."

(continues next page)

Box 3.5 Selected Medications Relevant to Nutrition Assessment of Eating Disorders[a] (continued)

In response, patients may inappropriately restrict intake and exercise excessively, behavior that can trigger an eating disorder in susceptible individuals. Such patients should instead be advised to use their prescribed medicine while they appropriately change behaviors to the point the medications are no longer needed.

- **Medications associated with increased appetite, impaired fluid excretion, or decreased metabolism**: Medication with the potential to increase appetite and/or weight can be scary for anyone who fears weight gain. This fear can lead a patient to underuse or disregard prescribed medications, or drastically restrict eating in an effort to counteract the medication's weight-related effects.
- **Medications that deplete nutrients or have known food-medication interactions**: Prescription of such medications should be accompanied by nutrition education.
- **Laxatives, enemas, diuretics, stimulants, and metabolic enhancers**: Not only dangerous on their own, these substances can also have potentially dangerous interactions with prescribed medications. Reduction of these substances should be medically supervised because they may have addictive effects in the gastrointestinal tract. Nonstimulant stool-softeners may be recommended as patients are weaned from laxatives. (See Chapter 9 for more detailed information about laxative abuse.)
- **Insulin**: Insulin is so often restricted to promote weight loss that it has spawned the name "diabulimia" (7). Eating disorders are twice as common among girls and women with diabetes who use insulin compared with females without diabetes. Women and girls who abuse insulin for weight loss have three times the risk of death from diabetes and its complications compared with females with diabetes who do not misuse insulin (8). Adolescents newly diagnosed with diabetes are considered to be a particularly at-risk group and should be monitored for abnormal weight loss, ketones, and high blood glucose levels. These findings may indicate dangerous manipulation/underuse of medication.

[a]See Chapter 8 for more information on medications.

DIET EXPERIENCE

The Food and Nutrient Administration category of nutrition assessment includes Diet Experience—the evaluation of the patient's past and present experiences with both prescribed and self-selected diets (1). Chronic dieting behavior and obsession with food can result in nutrient deficiencies, psychological stress, impairment in social functioning, excessive intake of bioactive substances, and other symptoms of eating disorders. Additionally, patients with a chronic dieting history may have accumulated many dieting "rules" that support their eating disorder. Investigating previous diets will provide you with a guide for your nutrition education and counseling.

Patients who are overweight may be discouraged by a history of unsuccessful attempts to lose weight or maintain weight loss through conventional means or "doing everything right." This frustration can lead to the harmful weight-loss attempts that precede and then trigger their eating disorder. In some of these cases, a patient cannot succeed with weight loss through appropriate means because he or she has an undiagnosed endocrine disorder (see Chapter 6). An endocrine consult is in order when a patient describes any of the following:

- *Gaining* weight while dieting
- Rapid weight loss or weight gain without a change in eating
- Abnormal appetite or cravings surrounding menstruation
- Lack of weight loss even though eating minimally and exercising

BEHAVIOR

As you investigate each patient's food/nutrition-related history, it is important to assess behavior, which is defined in IDNT as "patient/client activities and actions that influence achievement of nutrition-related goals" (1). The following sections identify some behavioral issues and explain their potential relevance to eating disorders.

BINGEING BEHAVIOR

DSM-IV and IDNT Criteria vs Patient Definitions of Binge Eating

"Binge eating" is defined in the DSM-IV as an excessive amount of food eaten "in a discrete period of time" accompanied by "a sense of lack of control" (2). The IDNT definition of "bingeing behavior" is "eating a larger amount of food than normal for the individual during a short period of time (within any two-hour period) accompanied by a lack of control over eating during the binge episode (ie, the feeling that one cannot stop eating" (1).

To meet DSM-IV criteria for binge eating disorder, binge eating must be accompanied by some of the following behaviors:

- Eating alone
- Feeling embarrassed by the amount of food eaten
- Eating much more rapidly than normal
- Eating until feeling uncomfortably full
- Consuming large amounts of food when not feeling hungry
- Sense of lack of control of overeating during the episode
- Feeling disgusted with oneself, depressed, or guilty after overeating

These are the "official" definitions of binge eating, but the word "binge" has many personal meanings for those who use it. A patient who tends to restrict his or her intake may consider any unplanned eating, or even a "normal" portion to be "bingeing." Do not restrict your assessment of binge eating to only patients diagnosed with bulimia or binge eating disorder as patients with anorexia also may experience and/or fear bingeing (2). Clarify what constitutes a binge episode for each patient, and avoid using the word "binge" when asking questions about food intake until you have confirmed that you understand how the patient is using the word.

Binge Eating Patterns

If possible, collect data on the times of day, types of food, and triggering situations related to a patient's binge eating. This information will guide your nutrition education and nutrition counseling interventions.

Food Choices and Nutrient Intake in Binge Episodes

Binge episodes typically include either "forbidden" foods that the patient intends to purge (eg, sweets) or low-calorie foods that the patient believes to be acceptable in large quantities (eg, lettuce). Regardless of nutrition content, binge eating in response to emotions is an eating disorder behavior.

Next Steps If You Identify Binge Eating Behavior

Binge eating is addressed with nutrition education and counseling, but it should also be evaluated by the mental health professional on the treatment team. In addition to being an end result of restrictive eating, binge eating can also be a symptom of depression, anxiety, traumatic stress, and/or other issues outside of the RD's scope of practice.

AVOIDANCE BEHAVIOR

IDNT defines avoidance behavior as "keeping away from something or someone to postpone an outcome or perceived consequence" (1). Eating disorder "rules" usually include avoidance of one or more foods, food preparation methods, and/or food groups. During nutrition assessment, ask which foods are avoided and why (see also Beliefs and Attitudes section, later in this chapter). During nutrition education and counseling, you will discuss these restrictions in more detail, determine which are valid restrictions (eg, due to food allergies or religious observance), and provide support for relaxing those restrictions that are not beneficial. (See Appendix A for information on restrictive eating styles.)

Avoidance behaviors may also include refusal to eat food prepared by others, refusal to eat food without looking up nutrition content, refusal to eat with other people or in public, refusal to eat foods of a specific texture, and refusal to attend social functions where food will be served. Avoidance behaviors should also be evaluated by the mental health professional on the team as they may be symptoms of anxiety, social phobia, obsessive-compulsive disorder, and/or posttraumatic stress disorder (2).

MEALTIME BEHAVIORS

Assess the patient's "manner of acting, participating, or behaving at mealtime" and how that behavior "influences the patient's food and beverage intake" (1). Inappropriate mealtime behaviors include frequent reheating of food over the course of a meal, inability to sit still for the duration of the meal, excessive cutting or mixing of food on the plate, crying or yelling during mealtime, drawing out the meal for an excessive period of time, and monitoring or criticizing what others are eating. These behaviors should be evaluated by the mental health professional on the team as they may be symptoms of anxiety, obsessive-compulsive disorder, attention-deficit disorder, or other issues. Also assess the mealtime behaviors of family members and significant others. They may report difficulties at mealtime, such as frustration with the patient and the patient's eating, attempts to force the patient to eat unwanted food, and/or irritation at the patient's food choices and behaviors. Share your findings with the mental health professional on the team who may consult with family members or with the patient and family together.

In inpatient and residential treatment settings, mealtimes with family members will be limited. However, in outpatient, day treatment, or transitional settings, family meals may continue. If the patient will be eating one or more meals each day with family members, include them when you provide your nutrition recommendations. Reinforce that a stable, calm environment for eating meals together is a requirement at this level of care. Ask family members to bring their mealtime concerns to you or another member of the treatment team, rather than addressing them to the patient during the meal. As recovery progresses, therapeutic meals under the supervision of the RD and/or other staff may be helpful in improving the mealtime experience for everyone involved.

Chewing and Spitting Food Out/"Sham Eating"

Chewing and spitting out food without swallowing (also called "sham eating"), excessive chewing of food before swallowing, and immediate regurgitation of food are all efforts to restrict energy intake. These practices have been reported in athletes who compete in weight classes and patients who have had bariatric surgery that limits their intake of food.

BELIEFS AND ATTITUDES

IDNT defines "beliefs and attitudes" about food as "conviction of the truth of some nutrition-related statement or phenomenon, and feelings or emotions toward that truth or phenomenon, along with a patient's readiness to change, food, nutrition, or nutrition-related behaviors" (1). Documenting each patient's beliefs and attitudes about food is an ongoing process that merely begins at the nutrition assessment. Eating disorder beliefs are often "unpeeled" like layers of an onion and only fully revealed over time.

Conflict with Personal/Family Value System: Food "Rules"

Our culture promotes many uses of food that are not related to hunger—food as a reward, withholding of food as a punishment, forcing children to "clean their plates" to earn dessert, and so on. Adults with eating disorders may perpetuate inappropriate food rules from their childhoods and may create additional rules, all of which impair their ability to nourish themselves.

Food rules that promote the eating disorder and/or inhibit appropriate eating will be addressed in detail during nutrition education and counseling. When eating disorder rules stem from family and/or religious beliefs, or when requirements for healthful eating contradict these rules and/or cause feelings of guilt or excessive wrongdoing, report your findings to the mental health professional on the treatment team.

Readiness to Change Nutrition-Related Behaviors

Assess each patient's initial readiness to change behaviors related to eating and nutrition. (See Chapter 10 for more information on readiness to change.) Note any of the following in your assessment:

- Denial of an eating problem in the face of evidence to the contrary
- Denial of the need for food for survival
- Refusal to consider recommended changes in eating
- Refusal to participate in the nutrition assessment
- Dishonesty in self-report of eating and other symptoms (ie, the self-report conflicts with records or documentation of intake by nursing staff)
- Diminishing the importance of recovery (eg, "I don't see why I have to give up my eating disorder. It's not hurting me.")

These internal barriers to change can hinder an accurate nutrition assessment, as well as nutrition education and counseling. Report your findings to the treatment team.

FOOD AND NUTRITION KNOWLEDGE

Nutrition-Related Information

Although individuals with eating disorders may seem to have immediate command and recall of infinite bits of nutrition minutiae, they usually demonstrate little ability to apply it correctly. Preoccupation about the calories and nutrient content in foods often results from anxiety and an effort to manage fearful thoughts of weight gain and loss of control. A hyperawareness of calories and certain nutrients in food and beverages can impair an individual's ability to eat normally and function.

Assessment of nutrition-related information will continue past the initial assessment and will guide nutrition education and counseling.

Food Preparation/Cooking

In inpatient and residential levels of care, knowledge of food preparation is not necessary, as all meals will initially be provided by the facility. In less-intensive levels of care, and as a patient prepares for discharge, assess the patient or caregiver's ability to prepare the foods included in the meal plan. Nutrition education and experiential exercises (grocery shopping, cooking, therapeutic meals) will address deficiencies identified in your assessment (see Chapter 9 for more information).

FOOD AVAILABILITY

In less-intensive levels of care, and as a patient prepares for discharge, assess the following aspects of food availability:

- Can the patient (or caregiver) afford foods needed to follow the meal plan?
- Does the patient (or caregiver) have access to food refrigeration and safe places to store and prepare food? Does the patient (or caregiver) have means of transportation or other means of obtaining foods needed to follow the meal plan?
- If the patient is a child or adolescent, is the caregiver willing and able to obtain and prepare foods needed to follow the meal plan on the patient's behalf?

The input of a social worker or other member of the treatment team familiar with local resources may be required to eliminate external barriers to recovery, such as lack of transportation to obtain food or financial need.

PHYSICAL ACTIVITY

The nutrition assessment includes the "level of physical activity and/or amount of exercise performed" (1). Additionally, ask patients if their level of activity is linked in any way to their food intake—for example, is physical activity used as a compensatory (purging) method. Refer to Box 2.4 in Chapter 2 (page 25) for suggested assessment questions. Information about physical activity will inform nutrition education (see Chapter 9).

Decreased or Sedentary Activity Level

Eating disorder behaviors that cause weight gain can also lead to "exercise resistance" (ie, an unwillingness to participate in physical activity). Exercise resistance can stem from bad past experiences related to physical education or athletics (eg, weight-related teasing, being forced to exercise to lose weight), mistaken beliefs about exercise (eg, "No pain, no gain!"), and/or fear of weight discrimination or ridicule while exercising.

Report your findings to the mental health professional on the treatment team. The RD can support the patient in seeking physical activities that are enjoyable, noncompetitive, and stress-reducing. (See Chapter 9 for more information on physical activity.)

Excessive Physical Activity Levels

In addition to excessive duration, frequency, and intensity of activities, other signs that physical activity is excessive include:

- Ignoring work, family, or other responsibilities to exercise
- Exercising against medical advice, or when injured or ill
- Refusing to take rest days
- Exercise-induced amenorrhea
- Diagnosis of multiple stress fractures
- Inability to meet the energy needs of exercise with intake

REFERENCES

1. *International Dietetics & Nutrition Terminology (IDNT) Reference Manual: Standardized Language for the Nutrition Care Process.* 3rd ed. Chicago, IL: American Dietetic Association; 2011.
2. American Psychiatric Association. *Diagnostic and Statistical Manual of Mental Disorders, Fourth Edition, Text Revision.* Washington, DC: American Psychiatric Association; 2000.
3. Setnick J. Micronutrient deficiencies and supplementation in anorexia and bulimia nervosa: a review of literature. *Nutr Clin Pract*. 2010;25:137–142.
4. Hatcher AS. *Nutrition and Addictions: A Guide for Professionals*. Chicago, IL: Behavioral Health Nutrition Practice Group of the American Dietetic Association; 2008.
5. Helfman BL, Dennis AB. Understanding the complex relationship between eating disorders and substance use disorders. *Renfrew Perspectives*. 2010;(Winter):2–4.
6. Fahy TA, Treasure J. Caffeine abuse in bulimia nervosa. *Int J Eat Disord*. 1991;10:373–377.
7. Mathieu J. What is diabulimia? *J Am Diet Assoc*. 2008; 108:769–770.
8. Goebel-Fabbri AE, Fikkan J, Franko DL, Pearson K, Anderson BJ, Weinger K. Insulin restriction and associated morbidity and mortality in women with type 1 diabetes. *Diabetes Care*. 2008;31:415–419.

Chapter 4

Nutrition Assessment of Anthropometrics, Biomedical Data, Medical Tests, and Procedures

INTRODUCTION

This chapter addresses nutrition assessment topics related to two categories in the International Dietetics and Nutrition Terminology (1): (*a*) Anthropometric Measurements; and (*b*) Biochemical Data, Medical Tests, and Procedures.

ANTHROPOMETRIC MEASUREMENTS

Relevant anthropometric data in the nutrition assessment may include the following:

- Current weight
- Current height
- Current body mass index (BMI)
- Recent weight change relative to usual body weight
- Highest and lowest body weights and the circumstances in which those weights occurred
- Body composition as determined by DEXA or other methods

Body Mass Index and "Normal" Weight Status

BMI is used in some facilities and by some health insurance companies as a gauge of weight status. A BMI less than 18.5 is considered to be the equivalent of less than 85% of standard, and therefore valid as a criterion for anorexia nervosa.

However, use of BMI for prediction of a healthy weight is limited, especially for adults, because it does not differentiate between males and females, or take into account body composition, muscle mass or wasting, loss of bone density, and other factors. Interpretation of BMI should be qualified by an assessment of the individual's personal characteristics and the clinical judgment of the registered dietitian (RD).

When assessing anthropometric data, be aware that eating disorders are at times misdiagnosed because of a pervasive misconception only the underweight can suffer from eating disorders. This is false. Patients with bulimia may have normal or slightly higher than normal body weights, and binge eating disorder can result in overweight or obesity. The RD should avoid making assumptions about eating disorder status based on weight categories.

Weighing Protocols

RDs and other staff members responsible for gathering anthropometric data should be trained in the special concerns of eating disorder patients. See Box 4.1 for suggested protocols for weighing patients.

Box 4.1 Weighing Protocol Guidelines

If a weighing protocol is not already in place at your facility, the following general guidelines can be used for training:

- Weigh individuals with eating disorders in private, apart from other patients and/or family members.
- Take time to discuss the data-gathering process with the patient beforehand, and, as much as possible, honor his or her preferences regarding when and how he or she will be weighed and measured:
  - Ask whether the patient prefers to be weighed in street clothes or a gown, and whether he or she wishes to be weighed at the beginning or end of the appointment.
  - Some patients may find it helpful (although they may be unwilling at first) to be weighed backward, or with their eyes closed, so that they are unable to monitor daily or insignificant weight fluctuations.
  - Patients whose weights are not in danger may prefer not to be weighed at all. You can advise them that (contrary to the messages conveyed by the American culture) frequent weighing is not essential to healthy weight maintenance.
- Use caution in sharing anthropometric data with patients. They will view every piece of information through the distorted "filter" of the eating disorder, and they may interpret "normal" or "healthy" values as upsetting or unacceptable.
- Do not discuss patient weights in group sessions even if a patient is comfortable with his or her weight, as the numbers and their inevitable comparisons may be triggering to other patients.
- Avoid comments, even compliments, about a patient's weight. "Good job! You gained a pound!" can trigger eating disorder thoughts and behaviors in a patient who has mixed feelings about this aspect of recovery. Statements like "But your BMI is fine!" will not comfort most eating disorder patients and may even reduce your credibility in their eyes.

(continues next page)

Box 4.1 Weighing Protocol Guidelines (continued)

- Discourage patients, family members, and staff from considering weight to be "good," "bad," or even a sign that the patient is "doing well" or "doing worse." Instead, treat weight as simply another vital sign, like heart rate, blood pressure, or temperature—one piece of information that is added to other pieces to paint a complete picture of the situation.
- Discourage staff and family members from commenting on weight as if it were something to be excited or disappointed about, since the patient cannot control his or her weight. Outside pressure on a patient to gain or lose weight can tempt him or her to manipulate it by water-loading or other means. It is acceptable to ask a patient how he or she feels about his or her own weight, rather than to say, "You must be so excited!" or "You must feel disappointed right now."
- Keep in mind that overweight patients may be just as obsessed with monitoring their body weight as underweight patients. Although family members may claim that an overweight patient "doesn't care" about his or her weight, this is unlikely.
- Encourage family members to strive for a "weight neutral" environment in the home, where eating, weight, and diets are not discussed. Family members and staff should not comment about their own weights in front of patients (or preferably at all).

"Ideal" Body Weight

Although it may not be prudent to share numerical weight goals with patients, you may need to estimate such targets for other purposes, such as facility or insurance records. The following points provide guidance for estimating weight goals:

- There is no universally accepted standard for computing "ideal body weight" for eating disorder recovery.

- Use available anthropometric data, facility protocol and the patient's weight history to inform your clinical judgment to estimate an initial weight goal.
    - This goal may be revised as the patient progresses in recovery and additional data points are available.
    - Keep in mind that it is impossible at the beginning of treatment to determine a single weight that will signify a return to health.
- Recent and past weight history provide helpful information for estimating healthy weight goals, but the pre–eating disorder weight should not automatically be the goal.
    - Many individuals develop eating disorders after appropriately initiating weight loss. In other words, their "usual" body weight was high, their current body weight is low, and their healthy body weight is somewhere in between.
    - Patients who were formerly very muscular but have lost much of their muscle mass should not be expected to return to their original weight in the acute recovery period.
    - Adolescents and even young adults who appear to have reached their maximum height may grow taller when nutritionally restored.

LABORATORY TEST DATA

Interpretation of "Normal" Test Results

Patients, family members, and inexperienced health professionals may interpret normal laboratory test results as evidence that intervention is not needed. However, laboratory test results in the normal range should be considered in the context of other information because laboratory data can be unreliable in reflecting the severity of an eating disorder (see Box 4.2) (2–4).

Box 4.2 Possible Reasons for Unreliable "Normal" Laboratory Test Results

- The patient's nutritional intake has declined over time, allowing for metabolic changes that maintain homeostasis.
- Although nutrient *stores* are depleted, blood tests that evaluate *serum* nutrient levels remain within normal limits.
- Dehydration increases volume-dependent laboratory values, allowing them to seem normal until the patient achieves normal hydration status.
- Vitamin and mineral supplements or consumption of fortified foods mask nutritional deficiencies.

Source: Data are from references 2, 3, and 4.

Laboratory test results become more accurate and useful once nutritional rehabilitation has begun. Therefore, nutrition assessment will need to continue over time.

Interpretation of Abnormal Test Results

Laboratory test results that are outside of the normal range are more meaningful to the nutrition assessment for eating disorders. Abnormal test values should be taken very seriously, as they usually indicate *severe* and long-term nutritional deficiency (2). (See Chapter 8 for more information on nutrient supplementation.)

Selected Relevant Laboratory Tests

Boxes 4.3 through 4.25 provide information about selected laboratory tests related to eating disorders and the information they add to the nutrition assessment.

Box 4.3 Laboratory Test: Albumin

- Albumin is an indicator of nutritional status.
- *Below-normal* albumin results from malnutrition, inflammation, shock, liver disease, Crohn's disease, and celiac disease.

Box 4.4 Laboratory Test: Amylase

- When either the salivary glands or pancreas are inflamed, amylase (a digestive enzyme produced mainly in salivary glands and pancreas) escapes into the blood. Salivary isoamylase levels are ordered when vomiting is suspected.
- *Above-normal* isoamylase results from vomiting; cholecystitis (gallbladder infection); infection or obstruction of the salivary glands (can be caused by vomiting); intestinal obstruction; pancreatic or bile duct obstruction; perforated ulcer; tubal pregnancy (may be ruptured); viral gastroenteritis; and macroamylasemia.
- *Below-normal isoamylase* results from damage to the pancreas; kidney disease; pancreatic cancer; and toxemia of pregnancy.

Box 4.5 Laboratory Test: Blood Urea Nitrogen (BUN)

- BUN evaluates kidney function, which can be compromised in severe cases of eating disorders and dehydration.
- *Above-normal* BUN results from dehydration; catabolism of somatic protein (eg, starvation); excessive dietary protein intake; impaired kidney function; decreased blood flow to the kidneys due to congestive heart failure; shock; stress; recent heart attack or severe burns; and obstructed urine flow.
- *Below-normal* BUN results from starvation; overhydration; and liver disease.

Box 4.6 Laboratory Test: Calcium

- Serum calcium levels are tied to albumin levels, not to dietary calcium intake.
- *Above-normal* calcium results from hyperparathyroidism and bone cancer.
- *Below-normal* calcium results from malnutrition; alcoholism; magnesium deficiency; vitamin D deficiency; and hypoparathyroidism.

Box 4.7 Laboratory Test: Complement C3

- Complement C3 is a sensitive indicator of nutritional status.
- *Above-normal* complement C3 results from cancer and ulcerative colitis.
- *Below-normal* complement C3 results from malnutrition, cirrhosis, hepatitis, chronic infections, and lupus.

Box 4.8 Laboratory Test: Creatinine

- Creatinine is an indicator of kidney function, which can be compromised in severe cases of eating disorders.
- *Above-normal* creatinine results from dehydration; muscle injury; impaired kidney function (can be caused by drug abuse); kidney stones; urinary tract obstruction; decreased blood flow to the kidneys due to shock; congestive heart failure; atherosclerosis; and complications of diabetes.
- *Below-normal* creatinine results from muscle wasting and pregnancy.

Box 4.9 Laboratory Test: Ferritin

- Serum ferritin is the most sensitive indicator of total body iron stores.
- *Above-normal* ferritin results from excessive iron supplementation; inflammation; liver disease; and hemochromatosis (iron storage disease).
- *Below-normal* ferritin levels result from inadequate dietary intake of iron.

Box 4.10 Laboratory Tests: Folate and Vitamin B-12

- Folate and vitamin B-12 are indicators of nutritional status and are also ordered to determine the cause of macrocytic anemia (when a CBC shows large red blood cells and decreased hemoglobin concentration).
- Deficiencies can cause altered mental status.
- *Above-normal* B-12 and folate result from pernicious anemia and liver dysfunction.
- *Below-normal* B-12 and folate result from malnutrition, alcohol abuse, vegetarian dietary intake, celiac disease, and Crohn's disease.

Box 4.11 Laboratory Tests: Hematocrit (Hct) and Hemoglobin (Hgb)

- *Above-normal* Hct and Hgb result from dehydration.
- *Below-normal* Hct and Hgb result from malnutrition and iron deficiency.

Box 4.12 Laboratory Test: Homocysteine

Above-normal homocysteine is related to folate and/or vitamin B-12 deficiency; atherosclerosis; homocystinuria; smoking cigarettes; chronic kidney disease; and risk of blood clots and heart disease.

Box 4.13 Laboratory Test: Iron (Fe)

- Serum iron is less sensitive than serum ferritin, but also an indicator of nutritional status.
- *Above-normal* Fe levels result from excessive iron supplementation or hemochromatosis.
- *Below-normal* Fe levels result from inadequate dietary intake of iron; vegetarian dietary intake; heavy or long duration of menstruation; pregnancy; rapid growth in children.
- Possible signs of iron-deficiency include headache, fatigue, and difficulty concentrating.

Box 4.14 Laboratory Test: Lipase

- Lipase can be an indicator of pancreatitis. The test is used to rule out pancreatitis after unintended weight loss.
- *Above-normal* levels result from pancreatitis and other pancreatic disease; kidney disease; salivary gland inflammation; bowel obstruction; and peptic ulcer.
- *Below-normal* levels may be an indicator of permanent pancreas damage.

Box 4.15 Laboratory Tests for Liver Function

- Alanine aminotransferase (ALT), alkaline phosphatase (ALP), and aspartate transaminase (ASP) tests evaluate liver function, which can be compromised in severe cases of eating disorders.
- *Above-normal* levels result from substance abuse (including alcohol, drugs, or steroids); malnutrition; and hepatitis.

Box 4.16 Laboratory Test: Magnesium (Mg)

- Magnesium levels can be an indicator of kidney and gastrointestinal function.
- *Above-normal* magnesium results from dehydration; laxative abuse; excessive use of over-the-counter antacids containing magnesium; hypothyroidism; and Addison's disease.
- *Below-normal* magnesium results from inadequate dietary intake of magnesium; diuretic abuse; laxative abuse; alcohol abuse; hypoparathyroidism; Crohn's disease; inflammatory bowel disease; celiac disease; surgery; burns; and pregnancy.

Box 4.17 Laboratory Test: Mean Corpuscular Volume (MCV)

- *Above-normal* MCV results from vitamin B-12 deficiency.
- *Below-normal* MCV results from iron deficiency; and thalassemia.

Box 4.18 Laboratory Test: Phosphorus (P)

- Phosphorus is an indicator of nutritional status.
- *Above-normal* phosphorous results from excessive supplementation.
- *Below-normal* phosphorous results from refeeding syndrome; vomiting; laxative abuse; diuretic abuse; alcohol abuse; thyroid disease; untreated diabetes; kidney disease; and malabsorption.

Box 4.19 Laboratory Test: Potassium (K)

- Tests for serum K levels are usually ordered during routine eating disorder evaluations.
- *Above-normal* potassium results from dehydration due to inadequate fluid intake; untreated diabetes; excessive intake of foods high in potassium; excessive potassium supplementation; tissue injury; Addison's disease; hypoaldosteronism; kidney failure; overuse of some medications (eg, NSAIDs, beta blockers, ACE inhibitors, and potassium-sparing diuretics); and incorrect processing of the blood specimen.
- *Below-normal* potassium results from refeeding syndrome; malnutrition; vomiting; dehydration due to diarrhea; acetaminophen overdose; hyperaldosteronism; abuse of over-the-counter diuretics ("water pills"); and normal use of some medications (eg, corticosteroids, alpha- and beta-adrenergic agonists, some antibiotics such as gentamicin and carbenicillin, and the antifungal agent amphotericin B).

Box 4.20 Laboratory Test: Red Blood Cell Count (RBC)

- *Above-normal* RBC may be an indicator of dehydration.
- *Below-normal* RBC may be an indicator of iron deficiency.

Box 4.21 Laboratory Test: Thyroid-Stimulating Hormone (TSH)

- Thyroid function may be abnormal due to an eating disorder, or predate it. Weight loss caused by thyroid dysfunction can mimic anorexia.
- *Above-normal* TSH results from starvation; hypothyroidism (acute or chronic); pituitary tumor; and inadequate administration of thyroid hormone when needed.
- *Below-normal* TSH results from hyperthyroidism; excessive administration of thyroid hormone when needed; and damage to the pituitary gland.

Box 4.22 Laboratory Test: Total Protein

- Total serum protein levels can be an indicator of nutritional status.
- *Above-normal* levels may be an indicator of chronic infections or HIV.
- *Below-normal* levels may be an indicator of inadequate dietary intake of protein; celiac disease; inflammatory bowel disease; kidney disease; or liver disease.

Box 4.23 Laboratory Test: Urine Output

- Urine output is an indicator of fluid balance.
- *Above-normal* urine output results from excessive fluid intake; psychogenic polydipsia; or inadequate sodium intake.
- *Below-normal* output results from dehydration (also evidenced by dark urine color); and abnormal kidney function.

Box 4.24 Laboratory Test: 25-Hydroxy Vitamin D

- *Above-normal* levels result from excessive supplementation.
- *Below-normal* levels result from inadequate vitamin D intake; inadequate fatty acid intake; lack of exposure to sunlight; malabsorption; liver disease; kidney disease; and normal use of some medications (eg, phenytoin, phenobarbital, or rifampin).

Box 4.25 Laboratory Test: Zinc (Zn)

- Serum Zn levels can be an indicator of nutritional status.
- Zinc deficiency can cause altered sense of taste, difficulty gaining weight, and symptoms of depression.
- *Below-normal* Zn levels result from malnutrition; inadequate zinc intake; and vegetarian dietary intake without zinc supplementation.

MEDICAL TESTS AND PROCEDURES

Electrocardiograms and Echocardiograms

An electrocardiogram (EKG) or an echocardiogram (ECHO) can reveal whether heart muscle and function have been damaged by the eating disorder. The nutrition assessment should include any dietary and/or physical activity recommendations made by the physician as a result of EKG or ECHO findings, such as bed rest or fluid restrictions.

Dual Energy X-Ray Absorptiometry

A dual energy X-ray absorptiometry (DEXA) scan can show whether the patient has normal (for age) or reduced bone density (osteopenia or osteoporosis). The nutrition assessment should include any dietary and/or physical activity recommendations made by the physician as a result of DEXA findings, such as calcium supplementation, exercise restrictions, etc.

REFERENCES

1. *International Dietetics & Nutrition Terminology (IDNT) Reference Manual: Standardized Language for the Nutrition Care Process.* 3rd ed. Chicago, IL: American Dietetic Association; 2011.
2. Yager J, Devlin MJ, Halmi KA, Herzog DB, Mitchell JE, Powers P, Zerbe KJ. *Practice Guideline for the Treatment of Patients with Eating Disorders.* 3rd ed. Arlington, VA: American Psychiatric Association; 2006.
3. Setnick J. *The Eating Disorders Clinical Pocket Guide: Quick Reference for Healthcare Providers.* Dallas, TX: Snack Time Press; 2005.
4. Setnick J. Micronutrient deficiencies and supplementation in anorexia and bulimia nervosa: a review of literature. *Nutr Clin Pract.* 2010;25:137–142.

Chapter 5

Nutrition Assessment of Nutrition-Focused Physical Findings

Nutrition assessment includes evaluation of "nutrition-related physical characteristics associated with pathophysiological states." The data may come from a nutrition-focused physical examination, interviews, or the medical record (1).

Physical symptoms of eating disorders vary from patient to patient, depending on duration of the illness, type of eating and purging behaviors, and general physical well-being. Visible physical signs of eating disorders related to malnutrition and purging are identified in the following sections. However, many patients will not show any of these signs. Patients with binge eating disorder or bulimia may seem physically "well" and at or above a "normal" weight. Patients with anorexia may not show visible signs of malnutrition until well into the course of their illness. Therefore the information presented here should be used as a guide, not as diagnostic tools.

EXTREMITIES, MUSCLES, AND BONES

Overview

Table 5.1 lists selected nutrition-related physical findings in the extremities, muscles, and bones.

Table 5.1 Physical Signs and Symptoms of Eating Disorders: Extremities, Muscles, and Bones

Signs/Symptoms	*Potential Association with Eating Disorders*
Arthralgia (joint pain)	Malnutrition
Bone fragility	Malnutrition, amenorrhea, inadequate calcium intake
Decreased body fat	Starvation
Acrocyanosis of hands and feet	Malnutrition
Frequent and prolonged injuries	Malnutrition, excessive exercise
Decreased muscle mass	Starvation
Chronic muscle soreness	Starvation, excessive exercise
Russell's sign (scars, scabs on knuckles)	Use of fingers to induce vomiting
Fatigue	Malnutrition
Changes in how clothes fit (specify)	Weight changes
Feeling cold all the time/ cold intolerance	Starvation
Peripheral edema	Malnutrition, inadequate protein intake, reduced cardiac function due to starvation

Changes in How Clothes Fit

Eating disorders are related to a disrupted sense of body size and shape, or "body image." For some patients, changes in the fit of clothes (or lack of change) are the only way they can identify a change (or lack of change) in body size or weight. Patients may have clothing rules or routines, such as trying on a certain pair of jeans to see whether they fit, or refusing to try on certain sizes of clothing when shopping. It is rarely helpful to insist to patients that they are not the size that they imagine they are. Body image can be so distorted that a patient may insist that clothing he or she is wearing must be mismarked, because it is impossible for that size to fit.

Cold Intolerance

If a patient reports feeling cold all the time, it may indicate a physiological adaptation to starvation. In starvation, body temperature decreases and adipose tissue normally used to produce heat and insulate the core is used for energy.

DIGESTIVE SYSTEM

Overview

Table 5.2 presents nutrition-related physical findings in the digestive system (mouth to rectum).

Table 5.2 Physical Signs and Symptoms of Eating Disorders: Digestive System

Signs/Symptoms	*Potential Association with Eating Disorders*
Constipation, abdominal distension/bloating, abdominal cramping, abdominal or epigastric pain, and/or excessive flatulence	Altered GI function, delayed gastric emptying, starvation
Diarrhea	Misuse of laxatives, altered GI function
Nausea, vomiting	Altered GI function, induced vomiting, misuse of ipecac
Blood visible in emesis (requires medical evaluation)	Esophageal damage or broken blood vessels from vomiting
Blood visible in stool (requires medical evaluation)	Constipation leading to hemorrhoids, misuse of laxatives
Reflux/gastroesophageal reflux disease	Preexisting condition or result of frequent regurgitation or vomiting

(continues next page)

Table 5.2 Physical Signs and Symptoms of Eating Disorders: Digestive System (continued)

Signs/Symptoms	*Potential Association with Eating Disorders*
Decreased sense of taste	Zinc deficiency
Ketone smell on breath	Inadequate carbohydrate intake
Oral lesions	Erosion by stomach acid during vomiting
Dry or cracked lips	Malnutrition and/or dehydration
Enlarged parotid glands	Vomiting, infection due to vomiting
Sore throat	Irritation due to vomiting
Damaged teeth	Erosion by stomach acid during vomiting

Appetite Level

A lack of appetite can be caused by a variety of factors, including certain medications, depression, traumatic stress, and so on. Patients with anorexia nervosa, however, may indeed experience hunger (see Box 5.1). Anorexia, the symptom, and anorexia nervosa, the disease, should not be assumed to go together.

Box 5.1 Feelings of Hunger and Eating Disorders

Our culture promotes the erroneous idea that "going hungry" is an effective, sometimes essential, weight-loss method. As a person becomes more starved, he or she thinks about food more of the day. In patients with eating disorders, this preoccupation can lead to fears of overeating. Patients with eating disorders may need frequent reassurance that eating when hungry does not cause excessive weight gain.

Taste Alterations

Zinc deficiency can lead to lack of sensitivity to taste and smell (2). Patients who report changes in taste—or a recent propensity to add salt, spices, or other flavoring to food—may be deficient in zinc. This deficiency may be more likely if the patient had been severely restricting intake or following a vegetarian eating pattern. (Overuse of condiments is not always related to zinc deficiency. It can also be a method of "ruining" food so that it is not edible.)

Nausea and Early Satiety

Both nausea and early satiety when eating can occur during nutritional rehabilitation. For patients who are accustomed to eating only tiny amounts, or to inducing vomiting after eating, food in the stomach can provoke physical pain along with the expected mental distress.

Patients who report physical discomfort during or after eating should be referred to the primary physician, who may be able to recommend prescription or over-the-counter symptom management. It is important to convey to the patient that GI discomfort must not be allowed to impede nutritional rehabilitation.

Diarrhea

Diarrhea can be related to eating disorders in many ways, such as the consumption of large amounts of refined carbohydrates in patients who binge; eating excessive amounts of foods known to induce diarrhea for the purpose of purging; or as a result of use and misuse of laxatives (among other possibilities). Diarrhea can discourage someone with an eating disorder from wanting to eat. Therefore, if diarrhea is noted in the nutrition assessment, refer the patient to a physician for evaluation.

Constipation

Constipation can be a result of eating disorder behaviors, including eating infrequently or not enough; "rebound" constipation after laxative abuse; inadequate fluid and/or fiber intake; excessive fiber intake; and laxative dependence. Constipation reported during the nutrition assessment should be evaluated by a physician.

Constipation can be inaccurately interpreted by patients with eating disorders as "bloating" or weight gain, which may discourage them from eating. In such cases, a nonstimulant laxative or other medication may be prescribed. If a patient has a history of laxative abuse, a supportive family member may be willing to hold the medication and distribute it as recommended by the physician.

Feeling of Food "Getting Stuck" in Throat

Patients with eating disorders may report difficulty swallowing or express fears of choking. This can be related to oral-motor issues; recent or past surgery of the throat, neck, or jaw; physical or emotional trauma related to the mouth or face; or simply a manifestation of anxiety about eating. Patients who report this feeling or fear during the nutrition assessment should be evaluated further by the medical and/or mental health professional on the team.

Oral Malformations and Infections

As with anything that impairs the eating experience or makes it unpleasant or uncomfortable, a cleft lip and palate, recent tonsillectomy, swollen glands, and so on can trigger food restriction and eating disorders. Any kind of mouth infection, pain, or sore or dental surgery can do the same. Oral sores can be caused by repeated vomiting and can become infected. Problems reported during nutrition assessment should be evaluated by the physician.

NEUROLOGIC, PULMONARY, AND CARDIOVASCULAR SYSTEMS AND VITAL SIGNS

Overview

See Table 5.3 for nutrition-related physical findings in the neurologic, pulmonary, and cardiovascular systems, as well as in vital signs.

Table 5.3 Physical Signs and Symptoms of Eating Disorders: Neurologic, Pulmonary, and Cardiovascular Systems and Vital Signs

Signs/Symptoms	*Potential Association with Eating Disorders*
Impaired concentration, neurological changes (eg, depressed, irritable mood)	Malnutrition
Arrhythmias	Starvation, misuse of ipecac
Dizziness, shortness of breath	Diminished cardiac function due to dehydration or malnutrition
Decreased blood pressure	Starvation
Dizziness upon standing from a seated position	Diminished cardiac function due to dehydration or malnutrition
Decreased heart rate	Starvation
Decreased body temperature	Starvation

Dizziness and Unexplained Falls

Fasting, long periods between meals, chronic undereating and/or dehydration can cause patients to experience dizziness upon standing or during exercise, fainting spells, and/or "blacking out." These can result from inadequate blood pressure response when standing from a seated position, a weakened heart muscle, and decreased blood volume.

Patients with eating disorders who report any of these symptoms should be evaluated medically and advised on appropriate physical activities (or restrictions) needed to prevent injury. Nutrition education and counseling will be provided regarding appropriate fluid and food intake, which eventually should normalize these symptoms. In the short term, bed rest, use of a wheelchair, intravenous electrolyte/fluid administration, and/or electrolyte-containing beverages may be recommended.

SKIN, HEAD, AND NECK

See Table 5.4 for nutrition-related findings you may observe in assessment of a patient's skin. Table 5.5 covers findings related to the head and neck.

Table 5.4 Physical Signs and Symptoms of Eating Disorders: Skin

Signs/Symptoms	*Potential Association with Eating Disorders*
Dry skin	Malnutrition, dehydration
Acanthosis nigricans (darkened skin)	Insulin resistance
Petechiae (broken blood vessels)	Vomiting
Scars on arms, legs, or midsection	Self-harm (cutting)

Table 5.5 Physical Signs and Symptoms of Eating Disorders: Head and Neck

Signs/Symptoms	*Potential Association with Eating Disorders*
Hair loss	Malnutrition[a]
Headache	Malnutrition[a], dehydration
Lanugo hair on face	Malnutrition[a]
Occipital wasting	Malnutrition[a]
Broken blood vessel in eye	Vomiting

[a]Possibly starvation-related.

REFERENCES

1. *International Dietetics & Nutrition Terminology (IDNT) Reference Manual: Standardized Language for the Nutrition Care Process.* 3rd ed. Chicago, IL: American Dietetic Association; 2011.
2. Setnick J. Micronutrient deficiencies and supplementation in anorexia and bulimia nervosa: a review of literature. *Nutr Clin Pract*. 2010;25:137–142.

Chapter 6

Nutrition Assessment of Client History

INTRODUCTION

Nutrition assessment includes information from the patient, family, treatment team, and medical records about aspects of the patient's medical and social history (1). A complete client history often emerges over several meetings. Client history data categories and their relationship to eating disorders are described in detail in the sections that follow.

SOCIAL HISTORY

The social history includes socioeconomic factors, housing situation, family and medical support, occupation, religion, history of recent crisis, and involvement in social groups, all of which may impact foods eaten and eating behavior (1). For the patient with an eating disorder, the following factors may be of particular relevance.

History of Recent Crisis (and Other Life Changes)

A divorce, a death, a marriage, a move to a new town or new school, a pregnancy or birth of a child, a child leaving home, a diagnosis of chronic or terminal illness, or more than one of these events at the same time can be overwhelming for anyone. Individuals with eating disorders are especially sensitive to changes like these that prompt altered routines, adjustments (even desirable ones), mixed feelings, confusion, or loneliness. In susceptible individuals, such changes can prompt a desire for weight loss, whether or not it is needed, and can trigger an eating disorder.

Recent life changes (or life changes that are not recent but were very traumatic) are important to the nutrition assessment because they may point to needs for nutrition education (eg, appropriate eating in the college cafeteria; cooking for two instead of four) and/or nutrition counseling (eg, nutrition needs of pregnancy and acceptance of pregnancy weight gain; eating even though appetite is decreased due to depression).

At times a connection between eating and a recent or past event may not be uncovered during the initial nutrition assessment. Whenever it surfaces, the registered dietitian (RD) helps the patient manage his or her eating, and the underlying stressor(s) should be referred to the mental health professional on the team.

Domestic Issues

A history of physical, sexual, or emotional abuse may influence a patient's body image, self-worth (including feeling "undeserving of food"), and tolerance of different foods/beverages or textures. Abuse and the lack of trust it can engender may lead to unwillingness to participate in nutrition counseling. Abuse can also lead to a conscious or subconscious dread of returning to a certain weight or body size. Learning to eat appropriately despite these issues is an earlier stage goal, and within the scope of practice for an RD. In contrast, learning to cope with the issues themselves can be a lifelong process, and is undertaken with guidance from a mental health professional.

The RD will typically read of a patient's history of abuse in chart notes, rather than hearing about this history directly from the patient. However, in cases where the

RD is the first member of the treatment team to learn of abuse, it should be reported to the mental health professional on the team.

Living/Housing Situation

A patient's living situation can play a huge role in development of and recovery from an eating disorder. Grocery shopping, food storage, and food preparation can be assisted or impaired by roommates, family members, and space constraints. Attending college may involve moving away from home for the first time, and can be a trigger for an eating disorder. Patients returning home from eating disorder treatment may also become responsible for their own grocery shopping and food preparation for the first time. Assessment of gaps in knowledge and skill will point to nutrition education and counseling goals.

Social Support

Nutrition assessment should include the availability of support for eating disorder recovery available from family members, loved ones and other caregivers. These supportive individuals should be included in some nutrition education and/or counseling sessions, especially if they will be present during meal times and/or the patient is a child or teen reliant on parents for obtaining food. Children with eating disorders are unlikely to go out of their way to eat, especially without supervision. Therefore, your time in the nutrition intervention may be most effectively spent with parents or other caregivers, providing guidelines for feeding, including appropriate portion sizes, food choices, timing of meals and snacks and mealtime behavior. The Maudsley approach is a treatment methodology based on training the family to change their behavior rather than focusing on the patient (2).

Occupation

Certain occupations (and some leisure time pursuits) can influence eating disorder behaviors as well as willingness to follow nutrition recommendations. Examples include careers that (*a*) provide little time to eat (eg, flight attendant, school teacher, emergency room worker); (*b*) rely on minimal body weight (eg, horse-racing jockey, lightweight crew); or (*c*) emphasize physical appearance over health (eg, model, actor, bodybuilder, fitness instructor, broadcaster). "Aesthetic" sports such as figure skating, gymnastics, and cheerleading may involve aspects of all three of these factors.

Nutrition assessment should include any reported connections between an individual's occupation or hobby and the eating disorder, such as the following:

- Maintaining weight below normal range to further career success
- Encouragement by others to lose weight below normal range to advance career
- A work schedule that precludes appropriate eating times/amounts or limits the ability to obtain food
- Excessive physical activity due to career demands, or physical activity without adequate time provided for appropriate nutrition
- Preoccupation with weight, shape, and eating due to demands of career on physical appearance

Religion

Certain cultural and religious practices (eg, fasting, food group restrictions) limit intake (see Appendix B). For individual patients, these practices can be related or neutral to the eating disorder. Nutrition assessment should provide context for religious eating practices—for example, was the patient religious prior to the onset of the eating disorder? Eating disorders, as well as schizophrenia and obsessive-compulsive disorder, can in some cases include a pathological pseudo-religious component (3). This can manifest, for example, as a fear that God will be disappointed or angry if the patient eats a certain food, or that something bad will befall the patient or another family member if religious food practices are not followed.

Nutrition assessment should include any religious beliefs that influence eating choices. If religious or pseudo-religious practices are medically contraindicated, alternatives should be discussed. Ideally, nutrition needs can be met within the preferred religious practices. However, many religions allow health concerns to override religious traditions when medically necessary. Consultation with a chaplain or other informed member of the patient's religion may provide helpful guidance.

NUTRITION-ORIENTED MEDICAL/HEALTH HISTORY

The nutrition assessment includes "patient or family member disease states, conditions, and illnesses that may impact nutritional status" (1). When investigating the family history, be aware that it may include diseases that the patient is trying to "avoid" (such as diabetes or heart disease) with restrictive eating practices.

The following sections identify some aspects of the patient's personal and family health history to consider.

RECENT MEDICAL EVENTS OR ILLNESSES

A medical diagnosis, psychiatric diagnosis, and/or condition requiring surgery can be extremely stressful for the individual and family members affected. Terminal diagnoses, as well as those that require a special diet, a change in eating habits, and/or a change in ability to care for oneself, can trigger or retrigger an eating disorder as well as concurrent depression.

For a patient with an existing eating disorder, an additional diagnosis or change in condition can be especially discouraging, leading to the fear that recovery is unattainable or "not worth it." This discouragement can affect a patient's willingness to meet nutrition-related goals. When a family member receives unpleasant medical news, stresses of care giving and fears of loss can trigger the eating disorder patient to practice eating disorder behaviors, either as a stress response or in an effort to restore a sense of control over the situation.

Involuntary weight loss, such as that caused by an illness or oral surgery, can also trigger an eating disorder in a susceptible person. Once the weight is lost, the patient may not want to gain it back, leading to restrictive eating. In other cases, an illness that requires someone to leave school or work, or miss a vacation or other event can lead to depression with its accompanying lack of interest in food.

Weight loss in a child or teen should always be evaluated for an emotional component. The nutrition assessment should include recent events as well as more remote events that were particularly traumatic for the patient, along with any known eating-related results.

OBESITY OR OVERWEIGHT

Childhood Obesity or Overweight

In addition to the fear of weight gain that is inherent in many eating disorders, a history of being overweight in childhood can lead patients to fear that they can maintain normal weight only through extremely restrictive eating. Because of the distortions also inherent in eating disorders, patients may believe that they were overweight when in fact they were not. Unrealistic standards set by family members, athletic coaches, or other authority figures may continue to influence a patient's self-perception well into adulthood.

Nutrition assessment should include the patient's recollection of childhood weight and eating history (to what factors does the patient attribute childhood weight gain?), as well as any information available from growth charts and family members that affirms or contradicts the patient's perception. Reports of teasing or punishment related to weight or eating can be as traumatic as other forms of abuse and should be relayed to the mental health professional on the treatment team.

Obesity or Overweight in Family Members

Patients whose parents were or are obese may excessively restrict their eating in a misguided effort to prevent their own obesity. Eating disorders develop, resulting in weight loss for some, but overweight for others—the very condition they had hoped to avoid. Weight issues in the family of origin can lead patients to believe that they are "destined" to be overweight.

Nutrition assessment should include any information reported about fears related to obesity being "genetic" or inevitable because these fears can influence the patient's eating and eating disorder behaviors.

PSYCHOLOGICAL DISORDERS

Bipolar disorder, depression, anxiety, schizophrenia, oppositional defiant disorder, attention-deficit disorder, obsessive-compulsive disorder, substance abuse and other mental illnesses can occur concurrently with eating disorders. Untreated mental illness may interfere with eating disorder recovery by impairing the patient's ability to follow recommendations.

Some of the medications used to treat mental illness have the potential to affect appetite and cause weight gain or loss (see Chapter 8). Such appetite and weight changes can trigger or exacerbate an eating disorder. Nutrition assessment should include medicines with nutrition-related potential as well as any reported adverse effects.

Family Mental Health History

Family mental health history—including addictions, eating disorders, depression, obsessive compulsive disorder, anxiety, and other mental illness—can be related to genetic susceptibility to eating disorders as well as learned behaviors, stress management, and coping skills. Although the exact genetic and neurochemical links are not yet fully understood, this information may provide a level of comfort to patients, helping them realize that their eating disorder is not their "fault."

Depression

Depression is common in individuals with eating disorders. The connections are not clear, but inadequate intake can lead to neurochemical disruption and depression, and depression can cause a lack of interest in food.

Depression related to eating disorders may improve with nutritional rehabilitation. However, depression should also be evaluated by the medical and/or mental health professional(s) on the team.

Anxiety Disorders

Anxiety disorders can occur concurrently with eating disorders, but the neurochemical links are not yet fully understood. Eating disorder behaviors may function as one way of reducing anxiety.

Ideally, the anxiety associated with eating will improve as the patient learns to tolerate anxious feelings and they eventually subside. However, in the short term, appropriate treatment for anxiety disorders is essential, since eating disorder recovery requires the patient to participate in anxiety-provoking behaviors, such as eating more than desired, or eating "feared" foods. Anxiety regarding eating and/or unrelated anxiety should be evaluated and treated by the medical and/or mental health professional(s) on the team.

Substance Abuse

Substance abuse (including abuse of alcohol) is often associated with eating disorders. Patients may use or have used cocaine, heroin, methamphetamines, or prescription stimulants in an effort to control their weight.

Many patients do not consider laxatives, diuretics, diet pills, or steroids to be substances of abuse. However, when used inappropriately or to excess, these medications can be as addictive and harmful as illicit drugs.

A hospitalized patient without access to chronically used drugs will begin to experience withdrawal. If a patient reports substance abuse (including alcohol) for the first time in the nutrition assessment, share this information with the other members of the treatment team so that the detoxification process can be monitored. Tremors can be a sign of withdrawal from alcohol. If you observe that a patient is experiencing tremors, this indicates a very heavy user who should be monitored during the withdrawal process. Medical staff should be alerted.

If a patient is physically or psychologically dependent on one or more substances, a weaning protocol under medical supervision may be required. Some substances can significantly increase or reduce a patient's metabolism, which will need to be taken into account during nutrition restoration.

Cognitive Impairment

Cognitive impairment may be significant enough to impact a patient's ability to follow nutrition recommendations. If cognitive impairment leads an individual to feel "different," "not good enough," or not accepted by peers, he or she may try to "fit in" by losing weight. In susceptible individuals, these weight-loss efforts can trigger an eating disorder.

Personality Disorders

Personality disorders—including narcissistic, borderline, passive-aggressive, avoidant, and obsessive-compulsive disorders—may be associated with eating disorders or simply occur concurrently (4). Many patients with personality disorders do not know this information about themselves, even if it is documented in the medical record.

The progress of patients with personality disorders in eating disorder treatment may be exceptionally slow, or it may take unexpected detours. This may manifest as ambivalence about recovery, suspicion of health professionals, or attempting to "befriend" the treatment team. In turn, you may experience feelings that surprise you—hopelessness, helplessness, frustration, irritation, or inadequacy—when working with such individuals. These are common reactions to working with a patient with severe personality issues. It is important that you are able to view these reactions as functions of the disorder, not evidence that you are ineffective as an RD. Discuss the specific situation with the mental health professional on the team to determine how to proceed. If the patient is not working with a mental health professional, review the case with a supervisor or trusted colleague. See Chapter 10 for more information.

CARDIOVASCULAR HEALTH

Nutrition assessment should include any heart condition that has special nutrition or fluid requirements, regardless of whether the condition is related or unrelated to the eating disorder.

Eating Disorder–Related Heart Damage

Eating disorders may decrease cardiac function. The patient might experience "skipping beats," shortness of breath, "heart pounding," chest pain during exercise, weakness, light-headedness, edema, or none of these. Any patient who has rapidly lost weight or has lost a significant percentage of body weight should be evaluated for cardiac stability by a cardiologist or other physician knowledgeable about eating disorders (5).

Personal or Family History of Cardiovascular Disease

Following a diagnosis of cardiovascular disease, patients are usually given recommendations to decrease intake of fat and saturated fat, increase physical activity, and so on. Some people without cardiovascular disease choose to follow a restricted diet in an attempt to avoid becoming the next casualty of a family history of heart disease. When combined with a predisposition to anxiety or a susceptibility to eating disorders, these dietary modifications may go to an extreme, such as attempting to eliminate all fat intake or other abnormal and unhealthy measures. This can be both the result and a trigger of an eating disorder, and can cause fear of following nutrition recommendations. Nutrition education and counseling can eventually address appropriate guidelines for heart health.

Counterintuitively, starving can cause cholesterol levels to increase. When this happens, patients may interpret their elevated cholesterol as "proof" that they must cut back even further. If their physician is not aware of the eating disorder, unneeded lipid-lowering medication may be recommended. In many cases, cholesterol will normalize with nutritional restoration.

ENDOCRINE/METABOLIC DISORDERS

Hormone abnormalities are not rare in the eating disorder population. However, they may be undiagnosed.

Diabetes, polycystic ovary disease (PCOS), hyper- and hypothyroidism, Cushing's disease, and other endocrine disorders can all interfere with an individual's ability to regulate weight. Males with eating disorders may have impaired testosterone levels. Appropriate diagnosis and treatment of hormonal/metabolic disorders are essential.

Hypo- or Hyperthyroidism

Hypothyroidism reduces metabolic rate, which can result in unwanted weight gain. This can lead to restrictive eating and an eating disorder in susceptible individuals.

Starvation can cause temporary hypothyroidism that resolves with nutritional rehabilitation. In some cases, hypothyroidism is permanent and requires life-long management.

Hyperthyroidism increases metabolic rate, which can result in involuntary weight loss. If a patient finds this weight loss desirable, hyperthyroidism can trigger an eating disorder.

Nutrition assessment should include any weight loss or gain unexplained by changes in eating.

Polycystic Ovary Disease

PCOS (also known as "chronic anovulation") results from insulin resistance. Signs and symptoms include difficulty maintaining a normal weight, carbohydrate and sweet cravings, and irregular menstruation (6). Severe acne, abnormal facial or body hair (distinct from lanugo), acanthosis, and/or skin tags can also be signs of PCOS. Although cystic ovaries (not the same as an ovarian cyst) are visible via a sonogram, some women with PCOS do not actually manifest the very symptom for which the condition is named. Instead, blood tests show abnormal levels of reproductive hormones and an abnormal insulin-to-glucose ratio.

Women with PCOS are often not aware of their condition, so they drastically restrict their dietary intake in an effort to lose or maintain weight. These restrictions can potentially trigger an eating disorder and discourage a patient from following nutrition recommendations involving increased intake.

Treatment for PCOS that normalizes insulin and other hormones can be beneficial to eating disorder recovery. Nutrition recommendations for PCOS are similar to recommendations for hypoglycemia. For more information, *The Dietitian's Guide to PCOS* (6) is recommended.

GASTROINTESTINAL CONDITIONS

Any diagnosis that causes gastrointestinal (GI) pain or requires a drastic change in eating habits can trigger eating disorders in susceptible individuals. Additionally, if a patient prior to diagnosis has experienced unexplained GI distress, he or she may have unnecessarily eliminated many foods attempting to find the source of the problem. Among the GI conditions to look for in the medical history are the following:

- Celiac disease
- Colon polyps
- Crohn's disease
- Diverticulitis
- Inflammatory bowel disease
- Irritable bowel syndrome
- Lactose intolerance
- Malabsorption
- Maldigestion
- Prolapsing hemorrhoids

Treatment and/or symptom management of any GI condition will be important because pain or discomfort during digestion will add to a patient's feelings of distress about eating. Nutrition assessment should include anything that impairs a patient's willingness to eat.

CHRONIC ILLNESSES

The stress of a chronic illness, especially one that requires extra focus on food, eating, and medication at mealtimes (such as diabetes, multiple sclerosis, or cystic fibrosis), can trigger rebellion in the form of restrictive eating. Missing school due to medical appointments, trips to the nurse's office, and other facets of these illnesses that lead a child or teen to "feel different" can also trigger eating disorders. Skipping medications to manipulate weight can give a false sense of control in a frustrating situation. Nutrition assessment should include any effects of chronic illness on eating.

Take note if the medical history includes chronic fatigue syndrome. The exact connection between chronic fatigue syndrome and eating disorders is unknown, but they occur concurrently in some cases.

FOODBORNE ILLNESS

Avoiding a food that once gave you food poisoning seems like a perfectly normal reaction. A patient with anxiety, posttraumatic stress, obsessive-compulsive disorder, and/or an eating disorder may react to fear of food contamination by avoiding an entire food group, all food not personally prepared, or all foods entirely. Nutrition education and counseling for such a patient may include information about the immune system's ability to fight contamination. Concurrently, fears and anxiety should be referred to the mental health professional on the team.

STRESS FRACTURES

Stress fractures are common in eating disorder patients who exercise against medical advice, exercise excessively, and/or have poor bone density. Refer to the physician for exercise recommendations/restrictions. Nutrition education and counseling may include information on calcium intake as well as other needs for bone deposition.

HYPOGLYCEMIA

Hypoglycemia is most serious in patients with diabetes. For others, it is uncomfortable and inconvenient, but not life-threatening until very severe.

Many patients with eating disorders experience symptoms of hypoglycemia, such as shakiness, irritability, fatigue and headache, as a result of long spans of time without eating. Some patients with eating disorders and hypoglycemia have learned through experimentation that symptoms respond to eating but are not aware that they can prevent the symptoms for the most part by eating more frequently or eating protein at each meal.

Hypoglycemia often resolves with nutritional rehabilitation. In some cases it pre-dates the eating disorder or becomes a permanent condition. Nutrition recommendations for hypoglycemia include protein at each meal, focus on whole grains and minimize concentrated sweets, and frequent meal and snack opportunities.

GYNECOLOGICAL CONDITIONS

Premenstrual Syndrome

For some women, the days before and during menstruation are accompanied by mood changes and food cravings. Patients with eating disorders may fear these food cravings as they might include "feared" foods. Education about the normalcy of these cravings and appropriate ways to manage them can help prevent binge eating or restrictive eating during this time. Symptoms of premenstrual syndrome, such as severe cramping or mood changes, should be referred to the patient's gynecologist or the physician on the team for evaluation.

Amenorrhea

Amenorrhea (absence of menstruation) can be a direct result of malnutrition. Other factors related to menstruation and eating disorders include the following:

- Women with eating disorders may have had irregularities in their menstrual cycles before the start of the eating disorder.
- Women with eating disorders who take oral contraceptives, whether for birth control purposes or to "regulate" menstrual cycles, may be unaware that they would experience amenorrhea if they were not on the medication.
- Some women with eating disorders continue to menstruate, without assistance from medication, even when they are extremely malnourished and underweight. Because menstruation has been so closely linked to eating disorder recovery, women in this situation may insist that they are healthy and do not require treatment for their eating disorder.
- Some women with eating disorders do not resume a normal menstrual cycle even after obtaining a normal weight and appropriate nutrition patterns.

In light of such individual differences, resumption of menses should not be considered an indicator of general health or the achievement of weight goals.

Because bone formation relies on adequate circulating estrogen, amenorrhea can lead to bone porosity. Hormone replacement therapy in the form of oral contraceptives is often prescribed to women with eating disorders who are not menstruating, with the goal of protecting bone mass and preventing additional bone loss. Research findings have been mixed as to whether this is an effective treatment for bone health in the absence of adequate nutrition (5).

TREATMENTS AND THERAPIES

Cancer Treatments and Therapies

Radiation therapy, chemotherapy, and medications used to treat or manage cancer can have adverse oral and GI effects. As a consequence, a patient's intake may be altered, and he or she may experience involuntary weight loss or nutrient depletions. Depression related to a cancer diagnosis and/or the difficulties associated with cancer treatment can cause lack of appetite. All of the above can trigger or retrigger an existing eating disorder.

Bariatric Surgery

As surgeries for the purpose of weight loss have become more common, the number of postsurgery patients in treatment for eating disorders has reportedly increased. It may be impossible to distinguish causes from effects. For example, which came first: The eating disorder or the weight problem? The weight problem or the depression? The eating disorder or the postsurgical weight loss? The eating disorder or the postsurgical complications? The eating disorder or the postsurgical weight loss and regain? Even if these questions cannot be resolved, gastric bypass, gastric banding, lap-band, gastric sleeve, and other weight-loss surgery should be considered a risk factor for eating disorders.

Surgery to Repair Athletic Injuries

When high-level athletes are injured, the inability to continue to compete can be devastating to their identity and self-esteem. While recovering from surgery to repair these injuries, they cannot consume the same amount of calories that they needed during training and competition without gaining weight. This weight gain (or the fear that such weight gain might happen) can trigger an eating disorder in a susceptible individual. Patients in this situation require nutrition counseling regarding their nutrient and energy needs for healing, and through the recovery process until normal exercise and eating have been resumed.

Oral Surgery

Oral surgery can impair the ability and desire to eat, and it may cause pain when chewing, swallowing, or both. Involuntary weight loss due to the inability to eat normally can trigger an eating disorder, or it may be welcomed by an individual with an eating disorder as an "excuse" to restrict.

Breast Augmentation Surgery

Individuals undergo breast augmentation for a variety of reasons, but those with severely distorted body image or body dysmorphic disorder may choose cosmetic surgery to "fix" imagined flaws or heal emotional wounds. Breast augmentation can also conceal the skeletal frame of a woman with anorexia, whose own breast tissue is minimal. Nutrition assessment should include any past or planned surgeries that may relate to a patient's body image or body acceptance.

Ostomy

The discomfort of an ostomy can reduce a patient's willingness to eat. Also, long-term or severe abuse of laxatives may lead to an ostomy.

REFERENCES

1. *International Dietetics & Nutrition Terminology (IDNT) Reference Manual: Standardized Language for the Nutrition Care Process.* 3rd ed. Chicago, IL: American Dietetic Association; 2011.
2. Lock J, le Grange D. Family-based treatment of eating disorders. *Int J Eat Disord.* 2005;37:S64–S67.
3. American Psychiatric Association. *Diagnostic and Statistical Manual of Mental Disorders, Fourth Edition, Text Revision.* Washington, DC: American Psychiatric Association; 2000.
4. Sansone RA, Sansone LA. Personality disorders as risk factors for eating disorders: clinical implications. *Nutr Clin Pract.* 2010; 25:116–121.
5. Yager J, Devlin MJ, Halmi KA, Herzog DB, Mitchell JE, Powers P, Zerbe KJ. *Practice Guideline for the Treatment of Patients with Eating Disorders.* 3rd ed. Arlington, VA: American Psychiatric Association; 2006.
6. Grassi A. *The Dietitian's Guide to Polycystic Ovary Syndrome (PCOS).* Philadelphia, PA: Luca Publishing; 2007.

Chapter 7

Nutrition Diagnosis

INTRODUCTION

This chapter surveys nutrition diagnoses that may be appropriate for patients with eating disorders. The most pertinent and urgent nutrition-related problem should be chosen for the nutrition diagnosis and phrased in the problem, etiology, signs and symptoms (PES) format (1–3).

The following sections use the organizational structure of the International Dietetics and Nutrition Terminology (3) to group nutrition diagnoses in three categories: (*a*) intake, (*b*) clinical, and (*c*) behavioral-environmental. The data presented here are a sampling; they do not encompass all possible problems, etiologies, or signs and symptoms that may be relevant to a specific patient with an eating disorder.

SELECTED NUTRITION DIAGNOSES: INTAKE

Box 7.1 Inadequate Energy Intake

Possible Etiologies:

- Diagnosis of anorexia nervosa
- Diagnosis of bulimia nervosa
- Disordered eating pattern
- Increased energy needs due to hypermetabolism
- Lack of interest in food due to depression
- Obsessive desire to lose weight
- Increased energy needs due to increased physical activity

(continues next page)

Box 7.1 Inadequate Energy Intake (continued)

Possible signs and symptoms:
- Failure to gain or maintain appropriate weight
- Fear of food
- Irrational beliefs about the effects of food on the body
- Restriction or refusal of food or energy-dense food
- Refusal of food due to fear of purging

Source: Data are from reference 3.

Box 7.2 Excessive Energy Intake

Possible etiologies:
- Diagnosis of bulimia nervosa, binge eating disorder, or eating disorder not otherwise specified (EDNOS)
- Disordered eating pattern
- Resolution of prior hypermetabolism without reduction in intake
- Overfeeding of parenteral/enteral nutrition
- Calories unaccounted for from IV infusion and/or medications

Possible signs and symptoms:
- BMI greater than 25 (adults)
- BMI greater than 95th percentile for age and sex (children and adolescents)
- Body fat percentage greater than 32% (women) or greater than 25% (men)
- Weight gain
- Intake of foods with high energy density and/or large portions of food/beverages

Source: Data are from reference 3.

Box 7.3 Excessive Oral Intake

Possible etiologies:

- Diagnosis of bulimia nervosa, binge eating disorder, or eating disorder not otherwise specified
- Disordered eating pattern
- Prior hypermetabolism without reduction in intake

Possible signs and symptoms:

- Weight gain not attributed to fluid retention or normal growth
- Intake of foods with high energy density
- Intake of large portions of food/beverages, food groups, or specific food items
- Binge eating
- Estimated intake that exceeds estimated or measured energy needs
- Highly variable estimated daily energy intake
- Conditions associated with a diagnosis or treatment, eg, obesity, overweight, or metabolic syndrome, depression, anxiety disorder

Source: Data are from reference 3.

Box 7.4 Inadequate Fluid Intake

Possible etiologies:

- Disordered eating pattern
- Increased fluid needs due to increased physical activity

Possible signs and symptoms:

- Acute weight loss
- Estimated intake of fluids less than requirements
- Plasma or serum osmolality greater than 290 mOsm/kg
- Elevated blood urea nitrogen (BUN) and sodium levels

Source: Data are from reference 3.

Box 7.5 Excessive Fluid Intake

Possible etiologies:
- Diagnosis of anorexia nervosa
- Diagnosis of bulimia nervosa
- Diagnosis of EDNOS
- Disordered eating pattern

Possible signs and symptoms:
- Estimated water and/or noncaloric beverage intake exceeding requirements

Source: Data are from reference 3.

Box 7.6 Inadequate Fat Intake

Possible etiologies:
- Diagnosis of anorexia nervosa
- Diagnosis of bulimia nervosa
- Disordered eating pattern

Possible signs and symptoms:
- Dermatitis (scaly skin) consistent with essential fatty acid deficiency
- Weight loss if insufficient calories consumed
- Impaired growth

Source: Data are from reference 3.

Box 7.7 Inadequate Protein Intake

Possible etiologies:
- Disordered eating pattern
- Diagnosis of anorexia nervosa
- Diagnosis of bulimia nervosa
- Food- and nutrition-related knowledge deficit

Possible signs and symptoms:
- Insufficient intake of protein sources compared with estimated needs
- Prolonged adherence to a very-low-protein weight loss diet

Source: Data are from reference 3.

Box 7.8 Inadequate Carbohydrate Intake

Possible etiologies:
- Disordered eating pattern
- Diagnosis of anorexia nervosa
- Diagnosis of bulimia nervosa

Possible signs and symptoms:
- Insufficient intake of carbohydrate compared with estimated needs

Source: Data are from reference 3.

Box 7.9 Excessive Fiber Intake

Possible etiologies:
- Diagnosis of anorexia nervosa
- Diagnosis of bulimia nervosa
- Disordered eating pattern

Possible signs and symptoms:
- Diarrhea
- Excessive flatulence
- Estimated fiber intake higher than tolerated or generally recommended

Source: Data are from reference 3.

Box 7.10 Inadequate Vitamin Intake (Specify)

Possible etiologies:
- Diagnosis of anorexia nervosa
- Diagnosis of bulimia nervosa
- Disordered eating pattern
- Increased nutrient needs due to prolonged catabolism

Possible signs and symptoms:
- Abnormal laboratory values [specify]
- Physical findings [specify]
- Estimated dietary intake of foods containing specific vitamins less than requirements or recommended level

Source: Data are from reference 3.

Box 7.11 Inadequate Mineral Intake (Specify)

Possible etiologies:
- Diagnosis of anorexia nervosa
- Diagnosis of bulimia nervosa
- Disordered eating pattern
- Increased nutrient needs due to prolonged catabolism

Possible signs and symptoms:
- Abnormal laboratory values [specify]
- Physical findings [specify]
- Estimated mineral intake from diet less than recommended intake

Source: Data are from reference 3.

SELECTED NUTRITION DIAGNOSES: CLINICAL

Box 7.12 Underweight

Possible etiologies:
- Disordered eating pattern
- Diagnosis of anorexia nervosa
- Excessive physical activity

Possible signs and symptoms:
- Body mass index (BMI) less than 18.5 (adults)
- Muscle wasting
- Decreased skinfold thickness and midarm muscle circumference
- Estimated intake of food less than estimated or measured needs

Source: Data are from reference 3.

Box 7.13 Overweight/Obesity

Possible etiologies:

- Diagnosis of EDNOS
- Disordered eating pattern
- Excessive energy intake
- Increased psychological/life stress
- Physical inactivity

Possible signs and symptoms:

- Body mass index (BMI) > 25 (overweight in adults)
- BMI > 30 (obesity in adults)
- BMI >95th percentile for age and sex (children and adolescents)
- Weight for height more than normative standard for age and sex (children and adolescents)
- Increased skinfold thickness
- Increased body adiposity
- Overconsumption of energy-dense food and beverages
- Large portions (more than twice the recommended portion size)

Source: Data are from reference 3.

SELECTED NUTRITION DIAGNOSES: BEHAVIORAL-ENVIRONMENTAL

Box 7.14 Disordered Eating Pattern

Possible etiologies:

Factors gathered during the nutrition assessment process that contribute to the existence or the maintenance of pathophysiological, psychosocial, situational, developmental, cultural, and/or environmental problems:

- Familial, societal, biological/genetic, and/or environmental-related obsessive desire to be thin
- Weight regulation/preoccupation significantly influences self-esteem

Possible signs and symptoms:

- Decreased cholesterol, abnormal lipid profiles, hypoglycemia, hypokalemia (anorexia nervosa)
- Hypokalemia and hypochloremic alkalosis (bulimia nervosa)
- Hyponatremia, hypothyroid, elevated BUN (anorexia nervosa)
- Urine positive for ketones (anorexia nervosa)
- BMI < 17.5, arrested growth and development, failure to gain weight during period of expected growth, weight less than 85% of expected (anorexia nervosa)
- BMI > 29 (EDNOS)
- Significant weight fluctuation (bulimia nervosa)
- Diagnosis of anorexia nervosa, bulimia nervosa, binge eating, EDNOS, or amenorrhea
- History of mood and anxiety disorders, such as obsessive compulsive disorder (OCD), depression, or personality disorders
- Severely depleted adipose and somatic protein stores (anorexia nervosa)
- Lanugo hair formation on face and trunk, brittle listless hair, cyanosis of hands and feet, and dry skin (anorexia nervosa)
- Normal or excess adipose and normal somatic protein stores (bulimia nervosa, EDNOS)

(continues next page)

Box 7.14 Disordered Eating Pattern (continued)

- Damaged tooth enamel (bulimia nervosa)
- Enlarged parotid glands (bulimia nervosa)
- Peripheral edema (bulimia nervosa)
- Skeletal muscle loss (anorexia nervosa)
- Low body temperature
- Inability to concentrate (anorexia nervosa)
- Positive Russell's sign (bulimia nervosa) callus on back of hand from self-induced vomiting
- Bradycardia (heart rate < 60 beats/min), hypotension (systolic blood pressure < 90 mmHG), and orthostatic hypotension (anorexia nervosa)
- Self-induced vomiting, diarrhea, bloating, constipation, and flatulence (bulimia nervosa)
- Always cold (anorexia nervosa)
- Muscle weakness, fatigue, dehydration (anorexia nervosa; bulimia nervosa)
- Denial of hunger (anorexia nervosa)
- Avoidance of food or calorie-containing beverages (anorexia nervosa; bulimia nervosa)
- Avoidance of social events at which food is served
- Fear of foods or dysfunctional thoughts regarding food or food experiences (anorexia nervosa; bulimia nervosa)
- Food and weight preoccupation (anorexia nervosa; bulimia nervosa)
- Knowledgeable about current diet fad (anorexia nervosa; bulimia nervosa; EDNOS)
- Fasting (anorexia nervosa; bulimia nervosa)
- Estimated intake of larger quantity of food in a defined time period, a sense of lack of control over eating (bulimia nervosa; EDNOS)
- Excessive physical activity (anorexia nervosa; bulimia nervosa; EDNOS)
- Eating much more rapidly than normal, until feeling uncomfortably full, consuming large amounts of food when not feeling physically hungry; eating alone because of embarrassment, feeling very guilty after overeating (EDNOS)

(continues next page)

Box 7.14 Disordered Eating Pattern (continued)

- Eats in private (anorexia nervosa; bulimia nervosa)
- Irrational thoughts about food's affect on the body (anorexia nervosa; bulimia nervosa; EDNOS)
- Pattern of chronic dieting
- Excessive reliance on nutrition terming and preoccupation with nutrient content of foods
- Inflexibility with food selection
- Misuse of laxatives, enemas, diuretics, stimulants, and/or metabolic enhancers (anorexia nervosa; bulimia nervosa)
- Excessive use of condiments and food mixing
- Diagnosis—eg, anorexia nervosa, bulimia nervosa, binge eating, eating disorder not otherwise specified, amenorrhea
- History of mood and anxiety disorders (eg, depression, obsessive compulsive disorder, personality disorders, substance abuse disorders)
- Family history of eating disorders, depression, OCD, anxiety disorders (anorexia nervosa; bulimia nervosa)
- Irritability, depression (anorexia nervosa; bulimia nervosa)
- Anemia
- Leukopenia
- Cardiac arrhythmias, bradycardia (anorexia nervosa; bulimia nervosa)

Source: Data are from reference 3.

Box 7.15 Excessive Physical Activity

Possible etiologies:
- Diagnosis of anorexia nervosa
- Diagnosis of bulimia nervosa
- Disordered eating pattern
- Irrational beliefs/attitudes about food, nutrition, and fitness

Possible signs and symptoms:
- Weight loss
- Depleted adipose and somatic protein stores
- Neglect of family, work, or other responsibilities to exercise
- Exercise exceeding levels needed to improve health or athletic performance
- Exercising when sick or injured, or in defiance of medical recommendations

Source: Data are from reference 3.

REFERENCES

1. Writing Group of the Nutrition Care Process/Standardized Language Committee. Nutrition Care Process and Model part I: the 2008 update. *J Am Diet Assoc.* 2008;108:1113–1117.
2. Writing Group of the Nutrition Care Process/Standardized Language Committee. Nutrition Care Process and Model part II: using the International Dietetics and Nutrition Terminology to document the Nutrition Care Process. *J Am Diet Assoc.* 2008;108:1287–1293.
3. *International Dietetics & Nutrition Terminology (IDNT) Reference Manual: Standardized Language for the Nutrition Care Process.* 3rd ed. Chicago, IL: American Dietetic Association; 2011.

Chapter 8

Food and Nutrient Delivery Nutrition Interventions and Pharmacotherapy

INTRODUCTION

Healthy eating is the foundation for all eating disorder recovery (1,2). Therefore, although nutrition diagnoses for individuals with eating disorders vary from patient to patient (see Chapter 7), the goals of nutrition interventions tend to be similar. Box 8.1 lists long-term goals appropriate for almost all patients with eating disorders, regardless of eating disorder type (3–7). Registered dietitians (RDs) play a role in each of the long-term goals, with their greatest impact in the areas of improved nutritional status and "normalized" eating.

Box 8.1 Treatment Goals for Patients with Eating Disorders

- Medical/physical stability and physical/nutritional health within parameters of age and concurrent medical condition(s).
- "Normalized" (ie, neither abnormally restrictive nor excessive) eating, including variety, balance, and nutritional adequacy; ability to modify eating when needed without experiencing intense feelings of guilt or wrongdoing; ability to separate self-worth from nutritional intake.

(continues next page)

Box 8.1 Treatment Goals for Patients with Eating Disorders (continued)

- "Normalized" (neither abnormally restrictive nor excessive) physical activity within health and fitness parameters, accompanied by appropriate nutritional intake for activity level; use of physical activity for enjoyment, stress relief, athletic training, and/or health and fitness, rather than as a compulsion, punishment, or compensatory method of purging of caloric intake; ability to include rest days without intense feelings of guilt or wrongdoing and to halt activity when injured or ill or otherwise recommended.
- Absence of compensatory (purging) behaviors, food rituals that interfere with eating, and self-harming behaviors.
- Healthy "coping mechanisms" (ways of dealing with stress) for stressors that formerly triggered eating disorder behaviors.
- Improved/stable mental health within parameters of concurrent mental health condition(s).
- Supportive social structure in place on an ongoing basis; ability to reach out to supportive family members/friends/peers for assistance when needed in order to prevent relapse during stress.

For most patients, you will identify multiple nutrition interventions and your primary challenge may be prioritizing them. Because a patient's ability to participate in eating disorder recovery depends on adequate nourishment to support coherent thought, nutritional stability is a priority above all other goals except for the patient's physical safety and medical stability (5).

This chapter addresses the first of the four nutrition intervention categories used in the Nutrition Care Process, food and nutrient delivery, as well as issues related to medication use. For information on nutrition education interventions, see Chapter 9. Nutrition counseling interventions are covered in Chapter 10, and Chapter 11 surveys the coordination of nutrition care.

THE EVOLVING ROLE OF THE REGISTERED DIETITIAN IN FOOD/NUTRIENT INTERVENTIONS

The RD's role in the treatment of eating disorders changes as recovery progresses (4). A severely ill patient in the initial stages of treatment is not likely to benefit from participation in meal planning; you should take on this responsibility at first. A medically well individual in outpatient treatment, on the other hand, might need very little guidance from you on exactly what to eat, but benefit from more education in portion sizes, observing hunger cues, and other nutrition topics covered in nutrition education (see Chapter 10). Even patients who typically manage their eating successfully may require more intervention from the RD when a new or stressful eating situation occurs.

MEAL AND SNACK PLANS

Considerations Related to Level of Care

A patient's ability or inability to meet his or her nutritional needs is a major factor in determining the appropriate level of care:

- In the higher levels of care (ie, inpatient, residential, day treatment), the patient may have little or no control over food choices or method of delivery, leaving the RD with most or all of the responsibility for diet orders and menus (5).
- In the lower levels of care (ie, intensive outpatient, outpatient), the RD may be limited to offering advice about food to the patient, while the patient bears

most or all responsibility for obtaining, preparing, and consuming food.

- As patients transition through levels of care, the RD and patient share meal planning responsibilities to varying degrees. Over time and depending on situational factors, patients may require more or less support from the RD. The progression from full reliance on the RD to full reliance on self is not linear. During stressful and/or transitional times, such as pending discharge from a treatment facility, the start and end of school semesters, or relocation, the RD may provide more structure for a patient who has previously been managing his or her own meal planning.

General Guidelines for Meal Planning

Boxes 8.2, 8.3, and 8.4 provide generalized guidelines for nutrition interventions for anorexia nervosa, bulimia nervosa, binge eating disorder, and eating disorder not otherwise specified (EDNOS). As with all nutrition interventions, dietary recommendations vary with each patient's nutrition assessment, nutrition diagnosis, and specific concerns. You may select the interventions that fit each patient's needs.

Box 8.2 Guidelines for Food and Nutrient Interventions for Anorexia Nervosa and EDNOS Similar to Anorexia Nervosa

- **Number of meals and snacks per day**: 3 meals plus 1 to 3 or more snacks depending on patient preference, facility protocol, and as needed to meet energy needs. (Note: If oral intake is not adequate to provide adequate calories, see Nutrition Support section, later in this chapter.)
- **Meal and snack timing**: Evenly spaced throughout waking hours; based on work/school schedule if appropriate. Times should be determined in advance and maintained as much as possible day to day. If appropriate, set time limits to prevent prolonged meals or insufficient time between meals, such as 10 to 15 minutes to complete a snack or 20 to 40 minutes to complete a meal.
- **Meal and snack content**: Small portions to start (such as 50 or 100 kcal more per meal than patient is currently eating), then advance as tolerated to meet energy needs. Use patient's preferences to start. Advance to meet macronutrient needs, then incorporate balance and variety as tolerated. Limit noncaloric condiments and nonnutritive sweeteners. Do not provide foods known to cause purging or other self-harming behaviors unless supervision is provided after meals.
- **Meal and snack supervision**: If appropriate, recommend patient have supervision while eating to support completion of meal and to discourage concealment or destruction of food. Patients may benefit from support after eating as well, in order to process feelings of distress and to discourage purging or other self-harming behaviors.
- **Meal- and snacktime behavior**: Discourage food rituals. Conversation should not focus on food.
- **Documentation of meals and snacks**: Document intake; have caregiver initial record if veracity of patient-generated records is questionable.
- **Beverage intake**: If patient has difficulty tolerating required food intake volume, limit beverage intake during meals. Limit caffeinated and/or noncaloric beverages. If patient complains of excessive thirst, evaluate medications and discuss with physician. If patient is dependent on caffeine, discuss weaning program with treatment team.

Box 8.3 Guidelines for Food and Nutrient Interventions for Bulimia Nervosa and EDNOS Similar to Bulimia Nervosa

- **Number of meals and snacks per day**: 3 meals and 0 to 3 snacks, depending on patient preference, facility protocol, and as needed to meet energy needs (Note: If oral intake is not adequate to provide adequate calories, or patient is unable to tolerate oral intake, see Nutrition Support section later in this chapter.)
- **Meal and snack timing**: Based on patient preferences and work/school schedule if appropriate. Times should be determined in advance and maintained as much as possible day to day. Avoid lengthy periods (> 4–5 hours) between meals/snacks. Patients who eat rapidly may benefit from a recommended goal for meal duration (such as 10 to 15 minutes to complete a snack or 20 to 40 minutes to complete a meal) and/or a 2- to 5-minute pause partway through a meal, to promote a slow, appropriate pace of eating.
- **Meal and snack content**: Small portions to start; then advance as tolerated to meet energy needs *without purging*. Include protein source at each meal, per patient preferences to start. Advance to meet macronutrient needs; then incorporate balance and variety as tolerated. Limit noncaloric condiments and nonnutritive sweeteners. Avoid foods known to cause reflux or indigestion. Do not include foods known to cause bingeing or purging or other self-harming behaviors unless supervision is provided after meals.
- **Meal and snack supervision**: Patients may require supervision to discourage purging or other self-harming behaviors after eating. They may also require supervision using the bathroom. Patients may benefit from support after meals to process feelings of distress. If meal preparation and/or clean-up trigger bingeing, delegate these tasks to others or provide supervision.

(continues next page)

Box 8.3 Guidelines for Food and Nutrient Interventions for Bulimia Nervosa and EDNOS Similar to Bulimia Nervosa (continued)

- **Meal- and snacktime behavior**: Discourage food rituals. Conversation should not focus on food. Address mindful eating and stress management before and after eating.
- **Documentation of meals and snacks**: Document intake, bingeing, and/or bingeing triggers. Patients may feel shame if food consumed in a binge episode is documented. If so, document only that a binge episode occurred. Document any compensatory behaviors.
- **Beverage intake**: If patient has difficulty tolerating volume, limit beverages at mealtimes. Limit caffeinated and noncaloric beverages. If necessary, limit carbonated beverages, which can be used to help induce vomiting. If patient complains of excessive thirst, evaluate medications and discuss with physician. If patient is dependent on caffeine, discuss weaning program with treatment team.

Box 8.4 Guidelines for Food and Nutrient Interventions for Binge Eating Disorder and EDNOS Similar to Binge Eating Disorder

- **Number of meals and snacks per day**: 3 meals and 0 to 3 snacks, depending on patient preference, facility protocol, and as needed to meet energy needs.
- **Meal and snack timing**: Based on patient preferences and work/school schedule, if appropriate. Times should be determined in advance and maintained as much as possible day to day. Avoid lengthy periods (> 4–5 hours) between meals/snacks. Patients who eat rapidly may benefit from a recommended goal for meal duration (such as 10 to 15 minutes to complete a snack or 20 to 40 minutes to complete a meal) and/or a 2- to 5-minute pause partway through a meal, to promote a slow, appropriate pace of eating.
- **Meal and snack content**: Modify as appropriate to meet energy needs. Include protein at each meal. Follow patient preferences as possible. Incorporate balance and variety as tolerated. Do not include foods known to be triggers for bingeing or other self-harming behaviors unless supervision is provided after meals.
- **Meal and snack supervision**: Supervise as needed. Patients may benefit from supervision or eating meals with others to encourage slow pace of eating, decrease of shame-based eating behavior, and social interaction. If meal preparation and/or clean-up trigger bingeing, delegate these tasks to others or provide supervision.
- **Meal- and snacktime behavior**: Discourage food rituals. Conversation should not focus on food. Address mindful eating and stress management before eating.
- **Documentation of meals and snacks**: Document intake, bingeing, and/or bingeing triggers. Patients may feel shame if food consumed in a binge episode is documented. If so, document only that a binge episode occurred.
- **Beverage intake**: Limit caloric beverages as needed. If patient complains of excessive thirst, evaluate medications and discuss with physician. If patient is dependent on caffeine, discuss weaning program with treatment team.

Meal Planning Methodologies

Note that Boxes 8.2, 8.3, and 8.4 do not list a standard *type* of meal planning method. This is because there is no single best way to structure a meal plan (4). To choose a meal planning method, refer to your facility's protocol (if applicable) and consider your patient's learning style, preferences, and need for structure.

If a patient has previously used a certain type of meal plan with success, you may consider using it as written (if it is still appropriate), or adapting that structure to the patient's current needs. In cases where a patient has used a meal plan in a destructive manner, you may choose to "start from scratch." Many options for meal planning have been created by facilities and RDs. Selected choices are summarized in Box 8.5 (8,9).

Box 8.5 Selected Meal Plan Options

- **Fully prepared meals**: eg, from an outside delivery service, a caregiver, or the facility's kitchen, based on meal pattern and dietary recommendations from the registered dietitian (RD) with little or no input from the patient.
- **Daily menus**: The RD or the patient with supervision of the RD writes out exactly what will be served at each meal/snack time, which is then prepared by the patient or caregiver.
- **Meal schedule only**: The RD or patient with RD supervision plans meal- and snacktimes; patient chooses from available foods at each time.
- **Daily food group goals**: A plan to eat a certain number of foods from each group each day, but no specific goals as to which foods are eaten at which times.
- **Meal schedule plus food groups**: A plan to eat a certain number of foods from each group at specific times of day.
- **Exchange lists**: see reference 8 for more information.
- **Calorie counting**: The RD provides a calorie goal for intake at each meal and/or each day, along with recommendations for how best to allocate those calories. Note: It is of course appropriate for the RD and hospital staff to document calories eaten in the medical record. However, because of the obsessive nature of eating disorders, patients can misuse calorie counting to promote restrictive eating and/or feelings of guilt or wrongdoing about eating. If a patient is already counting calories as part of his or her eating disorder, the RD, patient, and treatment team should decide whether to teach the patient a more holistic meal planning technique or instead make use of the patient's existing knowledge of calorie counting to support recovery.
- **The plate method**: see reference 9 for more information.

Food Variety/Choices

Individuals with eating disorders often report dividing foods into "good/healthy/allowed/safe" and "bad/unhealthy/not allowed/feared" categories. As the disease progresses, the latter group of "feared foods" may expand, leading to excessive restriction, compulsive overeating, feelings of guilt or wrongdoing, and/or compensatory behaviors when these foods are craved or eaten. Recovery often entails reintroducing many of these "feared foods."

The RD encourages patients with eating disorders to expand their palates and to be open-minded and factual about food choices, while taking into account that nutrition education alone may not be enough to change long-held beliefs, however incorrect they may be. Professional opinions differ on whether patients with eating disorders should be allowed to limit their food choices during the process of recovery or encouraged to eat those foods they specifically avoid. In a residential or hospital facility, patients can be coached through "food challenges," encouraged to venture beyond their eating comfort zones with a point or level system, and supervised after eating feared foods. In an outpatient setting, patients may be less motivated to take risks with food, and food challenges may have repercussions hours later, when patients are no longer under supervision. In many cases, the RD may actually recommend that a patient avoid challenging foods at the beginning of recovery and essentially "advance the diet as tolerated" in terms of risk. Such a patient may eat safe foods only until an adequate level of intake is reached. When an individual in outpatient treatment is considered ready and willing to take a risk with food, the RD or mental health professional on the team should develop a plan to help the patient avoid compensatory behaviors before or after the challenge.

Patients may need a long time to become flexible with food selection. In the short term, adequacy of energy and nutrient intake is the priority. It may not be very important which foods are used to meet these needs. If a patient's preferences, though limited, can provide for his or her basic needs, it may be appropriate to work within these preferences until the patient achieves greater comfort with food.

MEAL PLANNING VS INTUITIVE EATING

Your flexibility to offer more or less structure without judgment is a strength that will support your patient in feeling safe to ask for help when needed (4,10,11). Many patients are eventually able to manage their own meal schedule and decision making, maintain an appropriate body weight using their internal cues as a guide, and eat without excessive feelings of guilt or wrongdoing. This gold standard of recovery has come to be known as "intuitive eating."

The intuitive eating philosophy is described by Evelyn Tribole and Elyse Resch in their book, *Intuitive Eating* (12). Many RDs recommend this approach as a goal for patients with eating disorders, and modified versions of intuitive eating are taught in some eating disorder treatment facilities. In direct opposition to rigid diets with calorie limits and forbidden foods, intuitive eating encourages personally directed eating choices based on internal cues, enjoyable eating not motivated by guilt, and changing individual needs.

Individuals with eating disorders may be very excited to learn the principles of intuitive eating and want to use them right away to start eating without guilt and shame.

However, eating disorders impair the very abilities needed to develop intuitive eating—namely, awareness and willingness to honor internal hunger and satiety cues, regulation of internal emotional states, and acceptance of imperfection in eating. These patients must wait until further into recovery, after basic behavioral and nutritional parameters have been met (ability to eat a meal without compensatory behaviors, ability to eat several times per day, etc.), physical and mental stability has been restored, and cues (hunger, fullness, cravings, emotions) and responses (guilt, shame, regret, wanting more) have been practiced within the safety and structure of a meal plan (1,3). The following are reasons that individuals with eating disorders may not be ready to practice intuitive eating:

- Long-held habits and food rules are difficult to break, even when countered with accurate nutrition information.
- Patients have difficulty identifying internal cues such as hunger and satiety after years of ignoring these sensations. Appetite-related hormones such as leptin, ghrelin, cholecystokinin, adiponectin, insulin, and others may play a role (13–15).
- Patients who are able to sense hunger and satiety have difficulty honoring them, or honoring them before they are severe.
- Patients overrule internal cues with eating disorder rationale—eg, "I can't be hungry again so soon after my last meal."
- Anxiety about food and associated stress hormones interfere with the ability to sense hunger and satiety.
- Eating disorder symptoms such as early satiety, delayed gastric emptying, bloating, and nausea are misinterpreted as signs of satiety (3).

Eating solely in response to hunger and satiety cues, although a worthy goal, is not realistic for an individual in early stages of eating disorder recovery. As recovery progresses, the RD can use intuitive eating techniques to help patients learn to identify hunger and satiety cues *while still following a meal plan.* Patients can document their sensations of hunger and satiety alongside their intake, providing a record of whether or not those cues, if followed, would result in appropriate eating. Over time, the meal plan can be relaxed to allow for one or more decisions (what to eat, how much to eat, when to eat) to be made "in the moment" rather than planned in advance, and these choices can be reviewed by the patient and RD to determine whether the "intuitive" decisions were wise, or simply opportunities to practice the eating disorder.

In this context, it is important to note that meal planning for your patients with eating disorders is *not* diametrically opposed to intuitive eating. Meal planning is simply an earlier step on the path to intuitive eating for someone who has seemingly lost touch with his or her intuitive self. Both intuitive eating and eating disorder recovery require that the individual avoid dieting behavior, as it can lead to eating disorders in those who are susceptible (16). An eating disorder meal plan must differ from a "diet" in five essential ways:

- A meal plan created by an RD promotes both physical and mental health; it does not encourage weight loss at the cost of health.
- The RD's meal plan is (ultimately) intended to provide *adequate* calories, rather than calorie deprivation.
- The RD's meal plan is individualized for each patient, taking into account patient-specific goals and needs.

- The RD's meal plan can be modified and adapted based on input from the patient, as well as changes in needs and preferences and physical parameters.
- The RD's meal plan is a teaching tool, not a dogma. It is a stepping stone to independent choices, not a permanent goal.

MEDICAL FOOD SUPPLEMENTS

There is no consensus among treatment professionals for or against the use of meal replacement beverages, supplemental oral nutritional formulas, and other medical food supplements (puddings, shakes, etc) in the treatment of eating disorders. Patients differ in their attitudes toward supplementation as well. The following are among the responses you may encounter when recommending nutritional supplementation to meet energy needs:

- Some patients with eating disorders prefer food—their point of view is, "If I have to get the calories, I want to enjoy them."
- Others fear that if they eat and enjoy food, they will become overeaters. They prefer to ingest additional calories via supplements that seem more like medicine than food.
- Patients experiencing depression and an associated lack of interest in food may lack the motivation or desire to purchase, prepare, or consume regular food (17).
- Still others enjoy nutritional supplements, or enjoy the fact that supplementation is not "normal eating"—they are unwilling to give up the perceived cachet of having an eating disorder.

Supplemental nutrition, when acceptable to the patient, can be a useful tool to meet energy needs in excess of food intake (5,18). Supplements can also provide a balance of nutrients in situations where oral food intake is unbalanced or rigid.

To gain weight, many patients in treatment for anorexia require far more calories than might normally be expected (19–21). In these cases of hypermetabolism, where the energy cost of weight restoration is far higher than eventual (normalized) energy needs, a high-calorie liquid supplement can help meet additional calorie needs while the patient learns and practices eating a "normal" volume of food. Once metabolism has normalized, the patient can discontinue the supplementation while keeping food intake stable.

Experts debate how long a patient should be encouraged to use supplemental nutrition rather than meeting needs from food. Your facility may have guidelines regarding the use of supplemental nutrition at certain levels of care. If no guidelines exist, the RD may provide recommendations to the treatment team, and the decision should be made with the best interest of the patient in mind. Some patients need encouragement to transition from supplements to food; others wean themselves naturally as their recovery progresses. Certain individuals may continue to use supplements out of convenience, preference, or habit long after their other eating behaviors have normalized. If a patient is able to eat solid food when appropriate but chooses to use supplemental nutrition products when needed, there is no reason why he or she should be forced to discontinue their use.

NUTRITION SUPPORT

Nutrition support may be used in the treatment of eating disorders when it is medically appropriate and necessary. The RD has an important role in the initiation, monitoring, and advancement of enteral and parenteral feeding. At times, patients and/or family members may mistakenly view nutrition support as a punishment or use it as a threat to encourage compliance ("If you don't eat, you'll have to go to the hospital and be fed through a tube!"). The RD can assist by explaining the need for nutrition support and answering questions.

Enteral Nutrition

Enteral nutrition ("tube feeding") is an option for patients with eating disorders who are unable or unwilling to meet their energy needs with food or oral supplementation (22,23). If a patient is willingly refusing food and oral supplementation, a member of the treatment team should alert the patient that tube feeding is a next step. Knowing that tube feeding is imminent might motivate a patient to make a greater effort to eat. In other cases, the prospect of enteral nutrition can "reward" and reinforce aspects of the eating disorder (23).

Parenteral Nutrition

Total parenteral nutrition (TPN) and peripheral parenteral nutrition (PPN) are rarely used for patients with eating disorders because they do not support the healthful eating behaviors and hunger cues necessary for long-term recovery (5,22). When no other viable options exist for refeeding, TPN should be used for the shortest possible duration.

Indications for Use of Nutrition Support

Box 8.6 (5,6,22) summarizes possible indications for enteral and parenteral feedings for eating disorders. Refer also to Box 8.7 (page 127).

Box 8.6 Enteral and Parenteral Nutrition Interventions for Eating Disorders

Scenario 1

At each meal, the patient is offered a tray. Each time the patient refuses any oral caloric intake. *Intervention*:

- Initiate nasogastric (NG) feed with 30 mL isocaloric formula; increase as tolerated each feeding until required calories are provided.
- Each time the patient refuses oral intake, provide bolus feeding of equivalent calories.
- Do not tube-feed if the patient is willing to eat a full meal.
- Discontinue tube-feeding (remove tube) when the patient is willing and able to meet 90% to 100% of nutritional needs by mouth (all meals and snacks) for 48 hours.

Scenario 2

At each meal, the patient eats some food but refuses to finish the meal. Patient is offered an oral nutritional supplement equal to uneaten calories but refuses it.

Intervention:

- Initiate NG feed with 30 mL isocaloric formula; increase as tolerated each feeding until required calories are provided
- Each time the patient refuses to finish the meal, estimate remaining (uneaten) calories and provide bolus feeding of equivalent calories.
- Do not tube-feed if the patient is willing to eat a full meal.
- Discontinue tube-feeding (remove tube) when the patient is willing and able to meet 90% to 100% of nutritional needs by mouth (all meals and snacks) for 48 hours.

(continues next page)

Box 8.6 Enteral and Parenteral Nutrition Interventions for Eating Disorders (continued)

Scenario 3

The patient is eating but, due to poor appetite or fear of weight gain, cannot eat enough to prevent additional weight loss.

Intervention:

- Initiate nocturnal NG feed per facility protocol; increase as tolerated.
- Allow the patient to eat according to meal plan during the day. Subtract calories eaten from total needs and provide necessary additional calories continuously through the night until 3 to 4 hours before breakfast.
- Discontinue tube-feeding (remove tube) when the patient is able to meet 90% to 100% of nutritional needs by mouth.

Scenario 4

The patient is unable to think clearly, make competent decisions, or proceed in treatment due to malnutrition.

Intervention:

- Initiate continuous NG feed per facility protocol; provide total calories via 24-hour continuous drip.
- Once 100% of nutrient needs are being met, advance the patient as tolerated to bolus feedings at meal- and snack-times to promote normal pattern of hunger.
- Once the patient begins eating, subtract calories eaten from tube-feeding. Transition to nighttime tube-feeding if the patient is able to eat during the day.
- Discontinue tube-feeding (remove tube) when the patient is able to meet 90% to 100% of nutritional needs by mouth.

(continues next page)

Box 8.6 Enteral and Parenteral Nutrition Interventions for Eating Disorders (continued)

Scenario 5

The patient is eating but cannot meet the increased energy needs of hypermetabolism.

Intervention:

- Initiate nocturnal NG feed per facility protocol; increase as tolerated.
- Allow the patient to eat as possible throughout day. Subtract calories eaten from total needs and provide necessary additional calories continuously through the night until 3 to 4 hours before breakfast.
- Discontinue tube-feeding when metabolic rate normalizes and the patient is able to meet 90% to 100% of nutritional needs by mouth.

Scenario 6

The patient is medically unstable and, although willing to eat, cannot meet nutritional needs with food.

Intervention:

- Initiate continuous NG feed per facility protocol; provide total calories via 24-hour continuous drip.
- Allow the patient to eat as possible during the day, while increasing tube feeding to meet total energy needs. Once 100% of nutrient needs are being met via tube-feeding and oral intake, reduce tube feeding volume as oral intake increases.
- Discontinue tube-feeding (remove tube) once the patient is medically stable and/or able to meet 90% to 100% of nutrient needs by mouth.

Scenario 7

The patient has gastrointestinal (GI) dysfunction, such as involuntary regurgitation of food (gut rest not required).

Intervention:

- Initiate NG or naso-jejunal (NJ) feed, depending on the location of GI dysfunction; advance as tolerated to provide total calories via 24-hour continuous drip.

(continues next page)

Box 8.6 Enteral and Parenteral Nutrition Interventions for Eating Disorders (continued)

- Once GI function is restored, let the patient try a full-liquid diet, then progress as tolerated to small, easily digestible foods while providing additional needed calories via tube-feeding.
- Discontinue tube-feeding (remove tube) when the patient is able to meet 90% to 100% of nutritional needs by mouth.

Scenario 8
The patient has not met a goal weight or intake level previously established by the treatment team.

Intervention:
- Initiate tube-feeding (continuous, nocturnal, or bolus feedings); advance as tolerated.
- Tube-feed according to established plan.

Scenario 9
The patient is unable to meet energy needs via a combination of oral and enteral feeding.

Intervention: Supplemental peripheral parenteral nutrition.

Scenario 10
The patient requires total gut rest or cannot tolerate enteral feeding due to pancreatitis, GI blockage, or another medical condition.

Intervention: total parenteral nutrition (TPN).

Scenario 11
The patient sabotages or refuses oral and enteral feeding even when supervised.

Intervention: TPN.

Source: Data are from references 5, 6, and 22.

REFEEDING SYNDROME

When starved patients begin the process of nutritional rehabilitation, they can experience symptoms as their bodies readjust from the malnourished, metabolic "conservation" mode into a more normal utilization of energy and nutrients (24). These symptoms may be uncomfortable and annoying, such as flatulence, constipation, nausea, diarrhea, and bloating, or they may be dangerous and life-threatening, such as electrolyte imbalance and heart failure. These more severe symptoms as a group define "refeeding syndrome," which can be fatal.

Refeeding syndrome occurs when adaptations to starvation are rapidly reversed. Patients most at risk are those who weigh less than 70% of their usual body weight or have lost more than 10% of their body weight in the past 3 months (24). A patient's laboratory values may seem normal or near normal in the initial malnourished state (due to adaptations to starvation and dehydration). However, the patient's laboratory values may suddenly worsen when enteral or aggressive oral feeding begins. Careful, daily monitoring of phosphorous, potassium, magnesium, calcium and sodium levels, together with slow increases in tube-feeding volume, provide the best defense against such complications, especially during the first week of nutritional rehabilitation.

Box 8.7 (5,6,22) provides guidelines for initiating and advancing enteral feeding in a malnourished patient to decrease the risk of refeeding syndrome (25). At times, it may seem counterproductive to advance enteral nutrition at a slower than desired pace, but prevention of refeeding syndrome takes priority. Work closely with your patient's medical team to determine when it is appropriate to advance the tube-feeding rate, volume, and energy density.

Box 8.7 Enteral Feeding Guidelines to Decrease Risk of Refeeding Syndrome

- To protect lean body tissue despite a hypocaloric diet, begin protein repletion at 1.2 to 1.5 g protein per kilogram of ideal body weigh.
- Limit initial energy intake in accordance with intake during starvation. The infusion from the tube should not exceed 25 to 50 mL/hour. Rapid progression increases the likelihood of complications. Maintain client on a hypocaloric diet through the first 3 to 5 days. Then gradually increase calories toward full needs as tolerated. This may mean adjustments as minimal as 0 to 150 kcal/d until you are certain that tolerance is consistent.
- An isotonic, fiber-containing, polymeric formula is usually sufficient for nutritional repletion, unless impaired digestion or absorption indicates use of an elemental diet or peptide-based product. Maximize calories from fat and avoid high-glucose formulas.
- At initiation, limit carbohydrate to 150 to 200 g/d. Higher levels of carbohydrate exacerbate fluid intolerance. Monitor carbohydrate in the meal plan and the feeding formula until gradual and appropriate weight gain is established.
- Recommended fluid intake for the low-weight individual is 20 to 50 mL water per kilogram of body weight, or 1 mL water per kilocalorie of formula.
- Gradually increase the feedings by 10 to 25 mL/hour every 8 to 24 hours, if tolerated, until the target rate is achieved. Weaning can begin as soon as the tube-feeding objectives are being met and medical complications are resolved.
- During first week of enteral feeding, evaluate the following *daily:* body weight, blood glucose levels, fluid input and output, serum electrolytes, blood urea nitrogen (BUN), and serum creatinine levels.
- As enteral feeding continues and until levels are stable, evaluate the following *weekly:* serum prealbumin, calcium, magnesium, phosphorus, potassium, sodium, and creatine levels; BUN.

Source: Data are from references 5, 6, and 22.

VITAMIN AND MINERAL SUPPLEMENTS

Each patient with an eating disorder has a distinctive combination of eating practices, including food restrictions. When extreme, these practices can result in micronutrient deficiencies (see Table 8.1) Extreme restrictions can also lead to ingestion of abnormally large quantities of certain foods, or repeated intake of the same few fortified foods over and over again, resulting in excessive intake of micronutrients.

Table 8.1 Micronutrient Deficiencies Associated with Food Group Restriction

Restricted or Eliminated Food Group	*Potential Micronutrient Deficiency*
Dairy foods	Calcium, vitamin D, vitamin B-12
Vegetables	Potassium, folic acid, vitamin C
Meat, poultry, fish, and eggs	Iron, zinc, selenium, magnesium, copper, vitamin B-12
Fats, oils	Vitamins A, D, and E; essential fatty acids
Grains (bread, cereal, rice, pasta)	B vitamins
Fruits	Vitamins A and C, folic acid, potassium

Because nutritional issues vary from patient to patient, there are no standard recommendations for vitamin and mineral supplementation in eating disorders (4,26). Laboratory values often reflect long-term nutritional status rather than current intake, and can be misleading due to micronutrient supplementation. A thorough dietary history is more likely than laboratory values to indicate an individual patient's potential nutrient deficiencies.

Some eating disorder treatment facilities administer a daily multivitamin/mineral supplement to all patients admitted with eating disorders (4). This is an acceptable baseline to which additional single-nutrient supplements can be added on an individual basis. Table 8.2 (26) summarizes the available data on single-nutrient supplementation for patients with eating disorders.

Table 8.2 Micronutrient Deficiencies and Supplementation Guidelines for Eating Disorders

Nutrient	*Preferred Method to Assess Deficiency in Eating Disordered Patients*	*Eating Disorder–Specific Supplementation Guidelines*
Sodium	Serum Na < 136 mEq/L[a]	Refer to physician for prescription.
Potassium	Serum K < 3.5mEq/L[a]	Refer to physician for prescription.
Magnesium	Serum Mg < 1.5mEq/L[a]	Refer to physician for prescription.
Phosphorous	Serum P < 2.5mg/dL[a]	Refer to physician for prescription.
Calcium	Long-term—Poor bone density Short-term—Dietary inadequacy	Supplement with calcium citrate to total 1,500 mg/day elemental calcium from food and supplement; divide calcium dose into 500mg increments.
Iron	Plasma ferritin < 30 ng/mL for men, < 15ng/mL for women	Refer to physician for prescription; long-term administration and monitoring are necessary.
Zinc	Serum Zn < 46 ng/dL; hypogeusia (diminished sense of taste)	100 mg/day zinc gluconate (providing 14 mg/day elemental zinc).

(continues on next page)

Table 8.2 Micronutrient Deficiencies and Supplementation Guidelines for Eating Disorders (continued)

Nutrient	*Preferred Method to Assess Deficiency in Eating Disordered Patients*	*Eating Disorder–Specific Supplementation Guidelines*
Vitamin A (retinol, carotene)	Dietary inadequacy	700 mcg retinol/day for females >14 y of age (RDA); 900 mcg retinol/day for males > 14 y of age (RDA); supplementation above the RDA is not recommended
Vitamin B-1 (thiamin)	Dietary inadequacy; alcohol dependence	1.4mg/day (RDA).
Vitamin B-2 (riboflavin)	Long-term: activity coefficient of erythrocyte glutathione reductase > 1.4 Short-term: dietary inadequacy	1.3 mg/day for men (RDA); 1.1 mg/day for women (RDA).
Vitamin B-6 (pyridoxine)	Dietary inadequacy; alcohol dependence	1.3 mg/day.
Vitamin B-9 (folic acid)	Plasma folate < 3 ng/mL, or red blood cell folate < 140 ng/mL, or elevated plasma homocysteine	400 mcg/day.
Vitamin B-12 (cobalamin)	Serum B-12 < 200 pg/mL or elevated plasma homocysteine	1 mg IM cyanocobalamin/month or 2 mg oral cyanocobalamin/day.
Vitamin C	Long-term: 2-hour urinary excretion of vitamin C < 28 mg 4 hours after preload of ascorbic acid Short-term: dietary inadequacy	400 mg/day.

(continues on next page)

Table 8.2 Micronutrient Deficiencies and Supplementation Guidelines for Eating Disorders (continued)

Nutrient	*Preferred Method to Assess Deficiency in Eating Disordered Patients*	*Eating Disorder–Specific Supplementation Guidelines*
Vitamin D	Serum 25-hydroxy-vitamin D < 20ng/mL	No consensus.

[a]Note that abnormal blood values of these nutrients reflect long-term and/or serious whole-body deficiency. These should be medically evaluated and checked daily during the first week of nutritional rehabilitation because levels can decrease even with supplementation.

Source: Adapted with permission from Setnick J. Micronutrient deficiencies and supplementation in anorexia and bulimia nervosa: a review of literature. *Nutr Clin Pract*. 2010;25:137–142.

MEDICATION USE IN EATING DISORDER TREATMENT

Rationale

Eating disorder behaviors such as binge eating, self-induced vomiting, laxative abuse, fasting, exercising, and self-harm are thought to cause brain chemistry changes that relieve stress and balance brain chemistry. For some patients, the only way to stop the eating disorder behaviors is to provide a replacement medication, which may be required temporarily until healing has occurred, or permanently if needed.

The goal of psychoactive medications in the treatment of eating disorders is to promote improved brain chemistry. In rare cases, medications alone have been known to resolve eating disorder symptoms. For most patients with eating disorders, a combination of medications plus other treatment is required. By decreasing impulsivity, obsessions, anxiety, depression, and other psychiatric conditions, these medications do not instantly resolve eating disorder symptoms, but they provide a basic foundation from which patients can learn to change their habits.

Although the use of medication in the treatment of eating disorders is at times a trial-and-error process, it can be a hugely important and sometimes essential piece of the recovery puzzle. Once the eating disorder is in remission (generally defined as 6 months completely symptom-free), patients who would like to attempt recovery without medication can raise the issue with their physician. If the decision is made to decrease or discontinue a medication, all treatment team members (including the patient) should be alert for any symptoms or behaviors that may recur, as they may indicate a need for new behaviors, education, and/or return to medication.

FDA-Approved and "Off-Label" Uses of Medications

To date, the Food and Drug Administration (FDA) has not approved any medications specifically to treat anorexia, and only fluoxetine has been FDA-approved for bulimia (27). In clinical trials, topiramate has been studied as a treatment for binge eating disorder and bulimia, but it has not been FDA-approved for this purpose (28).

Once the FDA approves a drug for one condition, it may be prescribed for other "off-label" uses. Many medications originally approved to treat other psychiatric conditions are also used as treatments for eating disorders as well as underlying and concurrent disorders. When eating disorder patients are treated with appropriate medication(s) and dosage(s) by a skilled professional, their eating and mental symptoms may markedly improve or completely remit; however, for other patients, medications have no effect or produce adverse effects. Several medications may be tried before the best treatment is determined. Ideally, each patient works with a prescribing professional experienced with eating disorders who can monitor positive and negative effects and modify prescriptions as needed.

NUTRITION CONSIDERATIONS RELATED TO USE OF PSYCHOACTIVE MEDICATIONS

Many patients with eating disorders have been prescribed one or more psychoactive medications. Table 8.3 (5,6,27–31) summarizes the known potential nutrition-related effects and drug-nutrient interactions of commonly used psychoactive medications.

Table 8.3 Psychoactive Drugs with Nutritional Effects

Medication (Brand Names)	*FDA-Approved Uses*	*Potential Nutrition-Related Effects and Drug-Nutrient Interactions*
Alprazolam (Xanax)	Anxiety	• Decreased appetite and weight loss • Increased appetite and weight gain
Amitriptyline (Elavil)	Anxiety, depression	• Increased appetite, weight gain • Carbohydrate and sweets cravings • Increased blood glucose levels • High-fiber intake may decrease drug efficacy • Increased need for riboflavin
Amphetamine salts[a] (Adderall)	ADD, ADHD	• Decreased appetite and weight loss (can be dramatic) • Difficulty gaining weight

(continues on next page)

Table 8.3 Psychoactive Drugs with Nutritional Effects (continued)

Medication (Brand Names)	*FDA-Approved Uses*	*Potential Nutrition-Related Effects and Drug-Nutrient Interactions*
Aripiprazole (Abilify)	Depression, bipolar disorder, schizophrenia	• Weight gain • Constipation
Bupropion (Wellbutrin)	Depression, smoking cessation	• Decreased appetite and weight loss
Carbamazepine (Tegretol, Equetrol)	Bipolar disorder	• Decreased appetite
Chlorpromazine (Thorazine)	Schizophrenia, anxiety	• Increased appetite and weight gain • Increased serum cholesterol levels • Increased blood glucose levels • Increased need for riboflavin • Cardiac complications
Citalopram (Celexa)	Depression	• Weight gain
Clonazepam (Klonopin)	Anxiety	• Decreased appetite • Increased thirst • Weight gain or loss
Clozapine (Clozaril)	Schizophrenia, anxiety	• Weight gain (can be extreme) • Severe constipation • Cardiac complications • Increased blood glucose levels; new-onset diabetes mellitus • Increased serum cholesterol levels

(continues on next page)

Table 8.3 Psychoactive Drugs with Nutritional Effects (continued)

Medication (Brand Names)	*FDA-Approved Uses*	*Potential Nutrition-Related Effects and Drug-Nutrient Interactions*
Desipramine (Norpramin)	Anxiety, depression	• Increased appetite and weight gain • Sweets cravings • High-fiber diet may decrease drug efficacy • Increased need for riboflavin • Increased blood glucose levels
Dextro-amphetamine[a] (Dexedrine)	ADD, ADHD	• Decreased appetite and weight loss • Calcium or magnesium supplements may increase drug effect • Vitamin C supplement or acidic foods may decrease drug absorption
Doxepin (Simequan, Adepine)	Anxiety, depression	• Increased appetite and weight gain • Increased thirst • Sweets cravings • High-fiber diet may decrease efficacy • Increased blood glucose levels
Duloxetine (Cymbalta)	Depression	• Decreased appetite and weight loss • Increased appetite and weight gain
Escitalopram (Lexapro)	Depression	• Increased appetite and weight gain • Increased serum cholesterol levels

(continues on next page)

Table 8.3 Psychoactive Drugs with Nutritional Effects (continued)

Medication (Brand Names)	*FDA-Approved Uses*	*Potential Nutrition-Related Effects and Drug-Nutrient Interactions*
Fluoxetine (Prozac)	Anxiety, depression, bulimia	• Increased appetite and weight gain
Flurazepam (Dalmane)	Insomnia	• Decreased appetite and weight loss • Increased appetite and weight gain
Fluvoxamine (Luvox)	Obsessive-compulsive disorder, schizophrenia, panic disorder	• Decreased appetite and weight loss • Increased appetite and weight gain • Increased serum cholesterol levels
Lithium (Eskalith, Lithotabs, Lithonate, Lithane)	Bipolar disorder	• Weight gain • Increased thirst • Decreased appetite • Increased serum electrolytes • Bloating • Recommend noncaloric beverages and consistent sodium intake, limit xanthine (coffee, tea, cola)
Lisdexamfetamine[a] (Vyvanse)	ADD, ADHD	• Decreased appetite and weight gain (can be dramatic) • Nausea
Methylphenidate[a] (Ritalin)	ADD, ADHD	• Decreased appetite and weight loss (can be dramatic) • Difficulty gaining weight

(continues on next page)

Table 8.3 Psychoactive Drugs with Nutritional Effects (continued)

Medication (Brand Names)	*FDA-Approved Uses*	*Potential Nutrition-Related Effects and Drug-Nutrient Interactions*
Nortriptyline (Pamelor)	Anxiety, depression	• Increased appetite and weight gain • Carbohydrate and sweets cravings • Increased blood glucose levels • High-fiber intake may decrease drug efficacy • Increased need for riboflavin
Olanzapine (Zyprexa)	Schizophrenia, anxiety	• Increased appetite and weight gain (can be dramatic) • Can cause diabetes and/or ketosis • Increased cholesterol and/or triglycerides • Cardiac complications
Paroxetine (Paxil)	Anxiety, depression	• Increased appetite and weight gain (can be dramatic)
Pemoline (Cylert)	ADD, ADHD	• Decreased appetite (can be dramatic) • Weight loss or difficulty gaining weight
Phenelzine (Nardil)	Depression	• Increased appetite and weight gain • Phenelzine is an MAOI; limit high-tyramine foods

(continues on next page)

Table 8.3 Psychoactive Drugs with Nutritional Effects (continued)

Medication (Brand Names)	*FDA-Approved Uses*	*Potential Nutrition-Related Effects and Drug-Nutrient Interactions*
Phenytoin (Dilantin)	Seizures	• Decreased serum folate, phosphorus, calcium, and vitamin D levels • Decreased serum cholesterol levels • Increased blood glucose • Increased metabolism of vitamins D and K • Folic acid supplement >5mg/week lowers drug availability • Antacids, enteral feedings, and calcium supplements should be separated from drug administration by at least 2 hours
Quetiapine (Seroquel)	Bipolar disorder, schizophrenia	• Weight gain • Constipation • Increased blood glucose levels • Increased serum cholesterol levels
Respiridone (Risperdal)	Schizophrenia, anxiety	• Increased appetite and weight gain • Decreased serum sodium, hemoglobin, and hematocrit levels • Cardiac complications • Increased blood glucose levels

(continues on next page)

Table 8.3 Psychoactive Drugs with Nutritional Effects (continued)

Medication (Brand Names)	*FDA-Approved Uses*	*Potential Nutrition-Related Effects and Drug-Nutrient Interactions*
Sertraline (Zoloft)	Anxiety, depression	• Increased appetite and weight gain • Decreased appetite and weight loss • GI upset
Thioridazine (Mellaril)	Schizophrenia, anxiety	• Increased appetite and weight gain • Increased serum cholesterol levels • Increased blood glucose levels • Increased need for riboflavin • Cardiac complications
Thiothixene (Navane)	Schizophrenia, anxiety	• Increased appetite and weight gain • Increased need for riboflavin • Cardiac complications
Topiramate (Topamax)	Seizure disorders, migraine	• Decreased impulse to binge • Decreased appetite and weight loss • Increased lactic acid • Metabolic acidosis • Kidney stones
Trazodone (Desyrel)	Depression, insomnia	• Increased appetite and weight gain • Decreased appetite and weight loss • Anemia • Edema

(continues on next page)

Table 8.3 Psychoactive Drugs with Nutritional Effects (continued)

Medication (Brand Names)	*FDA-Approved Uses*	*Potential Nutrition-Related Effects and Drug-Nutrient Interactions*
Valproic acid (Depakote)	Bipolar disorder	• Increased appetite and weight gain • Increased serum cholesterol levels • False-positive ketones • GI distress • Polycystic ovarian syndrome • Altered thyroid function tests
Venlafaxine (Effexor)	Anxiety, depression, panic disorder	• Increased appetite and weight gain • Decreased appetite and weight loss
Zolpidem (Ambien)	Insomnia	• Binge eating or nighttime eating with amnesia, leading to weight gain

Abbreviations: ADD, attention-deficit disorder; ADHD, attention-deficit with hyperactivity disorder; FDA, Food and Drug Administration; MAOI, monoamine oxidase inhibitor.

[a]Due to their dramatic appetite-inhibiting side effects, these ADD/ADHD medications are potentially drugs of abuse among patients with eating disorders.

Source: Data are from references 5, 6, and 27–31.

The Role of the Registered Dietitian and Coordination of Care

The RD's role expands when a psychoactive medication is prescribed (29,30). Medication and nutrition influence each other, and medication efficacy may be enhanced or reduced depending on nutritional status. Not every patient will experience every adverse effect. However, the RD should be aware of the potential concerns and counsel the individual accordingly. In an outpatient setting especially, the RD may be the member of the treatment team most frequently in contact with the patient and may recognize that medication side effects are causing physical changes that patients attribute to eating more or to the consumption of certain foods. Appropriately ascribing these side effects, such as GI distress, weight gain, or decreased appetite, to medications and asking the patient to address them with the prescribing professional can improve the patient's willingness to continue nutritional rehabilitation (29).

Some patients and/or their family members express reluctance to use psychoactive medications, or even to simply meet with a psychiatrist. In these situations, it is important that your personal preferences and opinions regarding medication do not influence your professionalism. It is always appropriate to encourage the patient/family to bring any medication-related concerns directly to the prescribing physician, psychiatrist, or nurse practitioner, who can provide more information about the rationale for and risks and benefits of medication use.

If you are aware that a patient is noncompliant in taking medication (over- or underdosing, or use other than as prescribed) or is no longer taking a recommended medication, you or the patient should immediately report this to the prescribing member of the medical team, who can advise the patient.

If a patient self-medicates with either prescription medication or over-the-counter preparations, this should be reported to the psychiatrist or physician on the team, or a referral can be made if the patient has not had a psychiatric evaluation. Although self-medication (such as taking a friend's medicine) is inappropriate, it may indicate a legitimate need for medication.

Medication Use by Patients Who Self-Induce Vomiting

Patients who induce vomiting immediately or a short time after taking their medication may not receive the full effects of their medication. This should be addressed by changing the timing of meals, changing the timing of medication (with supervision of the prescribing professional), and/or behavioral intervention.

If a patient is abusing ipecac syrup as a means to induce vomiting, he or she should be counseled to stop immediately and the physician should be notified. Ipecac syrup builds up in the body and can be lethal.

Appetite-Inhibiting Medications

Medications with appetite-inhibiting side effects provide the greatest challenge for individuals who need to increase their caloric intake. Confer with the prescribing professional to determine whether the timing of dosage can be moved from before eating to after eating, or entirely separate from meal time.

Medications That Cause Weight Gain

Medications with the side effect of weight gain can be particularly distressing to individuals with eating disorders, regardless of their current weight. If a patient taking such a medication is at a healthy weight and gaining, overweight, or gaining weight rapidly without a concurrent change in eating, report the weight issue to the prescribing professional. In some cases, alternative medications can be prescribed. When there is no alternative medication, support your patient in following the meal plan rather than returning to eating disorder behaviors (29).

With medications that increase thirst or cause a feeling of dryness in the mouth, unnecessary weight gain can be mediated by reducing intake of calorie-containing beverages (31). Daily calorie intake may be dramatically reduced by a switch to water or other low-calorie beverages.

Other Adverse Effects

Encourage patients to report all adverse effects of medications to the prescribing physician, or contact the physician on their behalf. Even if adverse effects are reported, do not recommend that a patient discontinue a medication, as this is outside the RD's scope of practice. Some medications should not be discontinued without a weaning protocol, as they build up in the bloodstream over time.

Adjusting Dosages for Weight Changes

Certain medications are weight-dependent, and dosages may need to be adjusted when a patient experiences major weight changes. Report large weight changes over time to the prescribing physician.

REFERENCES

1. American Dietetic Association. Position of the American Dietetic Association: nutrition intervention in the treatment of anorexia nervosa, bulimia nervosa, and other eating Disorders. *J Am Diet Assoc.* 2006;106:2073–2082.
2. Gilbert SD, Commerford MC. *The Unofficial Guide to Managing Eating Disorders.* Foster City, VA: IDG Books Worldwide; 2000.

3. Tribole E. Intuitive eating in the treatment of eating disorders: the journey of attunement. *Renfrew Perspectives.* 2010(Winter):11–14.
4. Reiter CS, Graves L. Nutrition therapy for eating disorders. *Nutr Clin Pract.* 2010;25:122–136.
5. Yager J, Devlin MJ, Halmi KA, Herzog DB, Mitchell JE, Powers P, Zerbe KJ. *Practice Guideline for the Treatment of Patients with Eating Disorders.* 3rd ed. Arlington, VA: American Psychiatric Association; 2006.
6. Setnick J. *The Eating Disorders Clinical Pocket Guide: Quick Reference for Healthcare Providers.* Dallas, TX: Snack Time Press; 2005.
7. Kratina K. Health at every size: clinical applications. *Healthy Weight J.* 2003;17:19–23.
8. American Dietetic Association and American Diabetes Association. *Choose Your Foods: Exchange Lists for Diabetes.* Chicago, IL: American Dietetic Association; 2008.
9. American Diabetes Association. Create Your Plate. http://www.diabetes.org/food-and-fitness/food/planning-meals/create-your-plate. Accessed August 20, 2010.
10. Kellogg M. *Counseling Tips for Nutrition Therapists: Practice Workbook.* Vol 1. Philadelphia, PA: Kg Press; 2006.
11. Kellogg M. *Counseling Tips for Nutrition Therapists: Practice Workbook.* Vol 2. Philadelphia, PA Kg Press; 2009.
12. Tribole E, Resch E. *Intuitive Eating: A Revolutionary Program That Works.* 2nd ed. New York: St. Martin's Griffin; 2003.
13. Esterling E, Neubauer S. The relationship of ghrelin to appetite and weight management. *Weight Management Matters.* 2008;6(2):1–24.
14. Thomas S, Schauer P. Bariatric surgery and the gut hormone response. *Nutr Clin Pract.* 2010;25:175–182.
15. Bacon L. Tales of mice and leptin: false promises and new hope in weight control. *Healthy Weight J.* 2003;17(2):24–27.
16. Vredrvelt P, Newman D, Beverly H, Minirth F. *The Thin Disguise: Understanding and Overcoming Anorexia and Bulimia.* Nashville, TN: Thomas Nelson; 1992.
17. American Psychiatric Association. *Desk Reference to the Diagnostic Criteria from DSM-IV-TR.* Arlington, VA: American Psychiatric Publishing; 2000.

18. Tresley J, Sheean PM. Refeeding syndrome: recognition is the key to prevention and management. *J Am Diet Assoc.* 2008;108:2105–2108.
19. Moukaddem M, Bouier A, Apfelbaum M, Rigaud D. Increase in diet-induced thermogenesis at the start of refeeding in severely malnourished anorexia nervosa patients. *Am Soc Clin Nutr.* 1997;66:133–140.
20. Schebendach JE, Golden NH, Jacobson MS, Hertz S, Shenker IR. The metabolic responses to starvation and refeeding in adolescents with anorexia nervosa. *Ann NY Acad Sci.* 1997;817:110–119.
21. Salisbury JJ, Levine AS, Crow SJ, Mitchell JE. Refeeding, metabolic rate, and weight gain in anorexia nervosa: a review. *Int J Eat Disord.* 1995;17:337–345.
22. Caggiani C. Using enteral feeding to support eating disorder recovery. *SCAN's Pulse*. 1999;12–14.
23. Woods BK, Runyan B, Lamb RP. Perspectives in nasogastric feeding the eating disorder patient. *ICAN: Infant, Child, Adolesc Nutr*. 2009;1:257–261.
24. Tresley J, Sheean PM. Refeeding syndrome: recognition is the key to prevention and management. *J Am Diet Assoc.* 2008;108:2105–2108.
25. Caggiani C. Monitoring enteral feeding to support eating disorder recovery. *SCAN's Pulse*. 1999;10–11.
26. Setnick J. Micronutrient deficiencies and supplementation in anorexia and bulimia nervosa: a review of literature. *Nutr Clin Pract*. 2010;25:137–142.
27. FDA backs use of Prozac for bulimia. *New York Times*. November 13, 1994. http://www.nytimes.com/1994/11/13/us/fda-backs-use-of-prozac-for-bulimia.html.Accessed August 10, 2010.
28. McElroy SL, Arnold LM, Shapira NA, Keck, Jr. PE, Rosenthal NR, Karin MR, Kamin M, Hudson JI. Topiramate in the treatment of binge eating disorder association with obesity: a randomized, placebo-controlled trial. *Am J Psychiatry.* 2003;160:255–261.
29. Stein K. When essential medications provoke new health problems: the metabolic effects of second-generation anti-psychotics. *J Am Diet Assoc.* 2010;110:992–1001.

30. American Dietetic Association. Position of the American Dietetic Association: integration of medical nutrition therapy and pharmacotherapy. *J Am Diet Assoc.* 2010;110:950–956.
31. Pronsky ZM, Crowe JP. *Food Medication Interactions*. 16th ed. Birchrunville, PA: Food Medication Interactions; 2008.

Chapter 9

Nutrition Education Interventions

INTRODUCTION

The type of nutrition education you can offer a patient with an eating disorder will primarily depend on the treatment setting. In a general hospital or medical unit, nutrition education usually takes a backseat to food/nutrient delivery interventions (see Chapter 8), because most eating disorder patients only stay long enough to be stabilized and transferred to a specialty treatment facility or psychiatric unit. During a brief hospital stay, you may feel frustrated that a patient does not change his or her eating to follow your advice. Keep in mind that this is the nature of chronic illness, not a reflection of your effectiveness as a registered dietitian (RD).

Nutrition education in a short-term setting may be directed more toward caregivers and family members, answering questions and providing and/or recommending reading materials to help them understand their loved one's condition. If a patient is leaving your hospital for home, rather than an alternate treatment setting, provide a meal plan to the patient and/or caregiver that will be feasible in the home environment, along with a referral to an outpatient RD.

In treatment settings where you have multiple opportunities over time to gradually introduce and advance nutrition education, the topics you choose will vary depending on each patient's needs. Eating disorder patients may seem to know plenty of nutrition *information* (facts, Recommended Dietary Allowances, calorie counts), but most have little skill using this information to benefit their health.

Many of the nutrition "facts" that individuals with eating disorders use to guide their eating are unfortunately nutrition myths, misconceptions, or misinterpretations gleaned from magazines, peers, or even previous treatment experiences. In some cases, eating disorder practices are used to manage anxiety, even when the individual patient recognizes that these practices are not based on the realities of nutrition. Nutrition education for eating disorders, therefore, will likely focus on providing basic nutrition information to support better eating choices, the physical and nutrition-related effects of eating disorders and of nutritional rehabilitation, skills training to support nutrition recommendations (such as food shopping and preparation), and preparation for maintaining adequate nutrition after discharge.

NUTRITION EDUCATION PRINCIPLES FOR EATING DISORDER RECOVERY

If a patient has never previously encountered an RD, your first teaching topics will be the role you hope to play and the long-term nature of nutritional recovery. The information about your patient's beliefs and behaviors that you gathered during the nutrition assessment informed your creation of an initial meal plan. Because this initial meal plan might not have been nutritionally balanced, your patient or his or her family members may express concern that it does not reflect "normal eating." Reassure concerned caregivers that the initial meal plan is just a starting point for treatment, and, while it is impossible to predict at the beginning of treatment how long a full recovery will take, the eventual goal is eating behaviors and choices that are more balanced and appropriate.

The following basic principles of good nutrition provide a clear and logical framework for the path of nutritional restoration and show patient and family members how each step provides a necessary foundation for the next.

1. **Adequacy**: Intake during waking hours is sufficient to meet *energy* needs of daily living, voluntary physical activity, and weight goals.
2. **Balance**: Intake includes at least one selection from every food group and is sufficient to meet *macronutrient* needs.
3. **Variety**: Intake includes more than one food from each food group and is sufficient to meet *micronutrient* needs.
4. **Moderation**: Intake *does not exceed* recommended quantities of any food, nutrient, or bioactive or non-nutritive substance.
5. **Nutrient density**: Intake is *primarily* (not exclusively) composed of nutrient-rich foods.
6. **Calorie control**: Energy intake promotes *maintenance of appropriate weight* (or weight loss, if recommended).
7. **Autonomy**: Intake is based on *personal preferences* rather than the expectations of others. Nutrition factors—rather than weight concerns, obsessions, or irrational beliefs—are considered in planning meals. Regret after eating is manageable and does not result in compensatory behaviors.
8. **Confidence**: Intake is *spontaneous* and based on internal cues rather than a fixed schedule. Meals do

> not need to be planned in advance. Decisions can be made in the moment about what, when, and how much to eat. Participation in social and other activities does not revolve around what food will be available. Choices are almost always made without regret.

The principles build on each other, prioritizing necessities and presenting a new challenge as each goal is met. Therefore, they must be adopted sequentially to provide a solid foundation for long-term recovery.

Consider a patient whose meal plan includes eating scrambled eggs several times each day. You can use the principles of good nutrition for eating disorder recovery to help concerned family members understand that the patient is striving to eat *adequate* calories and that scrambled eggs are one of the few "safe" foods that he or she will eat in a large enough quantity to do so. With your gentle guidance and support, the family learns that scrambled eggs are only the first step in a comprehensive plan to move the patient toward health and confidence.

A patient may fear reaching the confidence stage because he or she believes that this final step requires giving up all control over food. Reassure your patient that this stage actually signifies being *in* control of eating and food rather than being controlled *by* them. Confidence is the intersection of good nutrition and internally guided eating. A patient in the confidence stage of recovery does not eat "anything and everything" indiscriminately. Instead, he or she makes choices based on appropriate criteria (hunger level, food availability, likes and dislikes, to name a few) rather than fear. This is also helpful information for family members, who may mistake personal choices (such as declining dessert) for eating disorder behavior.

"LEGALIZING" FOOD

Education that individual foods are not inherently "good" or "bad" is essential for eating disorder patients attempting to avoid compensatory behaviors caused by overwhelming feelings of guilt or wrongdoing after eating (1). *Legalizing food* describes the process of "decriminalizing" eating and removing moral qualities and "magical" powers from food. Individuals retain their preferences and autonomy in making food choices, but food returns to its appropriate status as simply (but so importantly!) nourishment for life. Foods are no longer referred to as "good" and "bad," but "more nutritious" or "less nutritious"; "more to my liking" or "less to my liking"; "locally grown"; "organically farmed"; "supportive to my recovery"; and so on. Legalizing a food does not mean the food *must* be eaten; it only means that the food *can* be eaten without guilt or shame.

The important distinction between an appropriate food restriction and an eating disordered one is the rationale behind the restriction. Individuals who have restricted themselves from eating some or many foods may need to learn again which foods they actually like and dislike outside of the context of food rules or fears. Recovery presents an opportunity to re-create food and beverage preferences—to try different choices and determine which to include in daily life and which to include only occasionally

Legalizing food does not happen in one fell swoop. However, as this policy is adopted over time, it neutralizes the power of "forbidden" or "fear" foods (2). When foods no longer have the ability to make the eater "good" or "bad," feelings of wrongdoing decrease, along with compensatory measures and overeating.

Nutrition education in eating disorder recovery can include the concept of legalizing food, even before it is realistic as a goal or behavior. Patients may have days or weeks of therapeutic eating experiences before they can eat a formerly forbidden food without remorse. Because American culture reinforces the "good/bad" dichotomy of food, patients will be challenged by external messages at the same time you are helping them change their internal ones.

If your facility encourages or requires patients to eat "risk" foods or "food challenges," or if you do this in an outpatient setting, support the participants in making plans in advance to manage the intense feelings of guilt and wrongdoing that may arise, along with the temptations to purge. Help educate patients that guilt experienced after eating food, or enjoying eating food, is not caused by the food itself but by an individual's internal beliefs about the food. These beliefs are flexible and can be altered, changing the experience of eating to an acceptable—perhaps eventually enjoyable—part of life, rather than something to be avoided or regretted.

WEIGHT GOALS

Weight is a compelling issue for many parties during eating disorder treatment:

- Patients are often desperate to know what you think their weight should be, how fast they will be expected to gain weight, how quickly they can possibly lose weight, and even how their appearance will change with their weight.
- Family members may use weight restoration as the hallmark of recovery and prefer weight normalization at any cost rather than well-rounded treatment.

- Insurance companies may use weight information as the sole determining factor for coverage decisions.

However, discussions about weight goals can distract from the true work of recovery. Educate your patients that "ideal body weight" is a concept, not a single fixed number for each person. Explain that a truly healthy weight is one that can be maintained with appropriate eating and physical activity, without purging or other eating disorder behaviors, and one at which vital functions (such as blood pressure, body temperature, heart rate, and reproductive functioning) are within normal limits. This healthy weight will be a *result* of eating disorder recovery, not its goal.

As much as possible, avoid lengthy discussions of weight-related numbers with patients, including future weight goals, current weight, body mass index, and weight changes. Patients may enter treatment with "fear" weights in mind, and they may already be or may become obsessed with certain body weights.

Fear of a certain weight may be linked to many factors, such as past experiences at that weight; recommended weight goals previously made by family members, medical professionals, Web sites, or other sources; comparison with friends, family members, or celebrities; or simply how a person imagines he or she would look at that weight. Patients may also fear that reaching a goal weight will signify that they no longer need the support of treatment professionals and family members, and try to sabotage their recovery to "stay sick" and therefore stay in treatment.

When you learn that a patient has a fear of a specific weight, or a fear of recovery in general, encourage the patient to share this information with the mental health professional on the team. Occasionally, family members will attempt to sabotage a patient's recovery because of their *own* fears—"If she gets better, she'll leave because she won't need me any more"—or their disagreement with recommended weight goals. If you believe that this is happening, share what you have observed with the family therapist or other mental health professional on the team who can address these concerns.

WEIGHT CHANGES

Patients and their families may benefit from education about weight changes during recovery. Box 9.1 summarizes the American Psychiatric Association guidelines for rate of weight gain in inpatient and outpatient care (3) and includes suggestions for facility-specific objectives.

Box 9.1 Guidelines for Rate of Weight Gain or Loss in Eating Disorder Treatment

The following basic recommendations should be modified depending on each patient's needs. Modify meal plans on an individual basis by monitoring the pace of weight changes. Once a patient has reached an appropriate level of energy intake, change meal plans based on a pattern of data, rather than on a daily basis.

Weight Gain Guidelines

- In higher levels of care, such as inpatient or residential treatment, more rapid weight gain can be expected and monitored than in less intensive levels of care.
- American Psychiatric Association Practice (APA) Guidelines (3) suggest 2 to 3 pounds of weight gain per week when an eating disorder patient is underweight at the start of treatment. Some treatment center protocols strive for 3 to 5 pounds of weight gain weekly.

(continues next page)

Box 9.1 Guidelines for Rate of Weight Gain or Loss in Eating Disorder Treatment (continued)

- APA Practice Guidelines suggest 0.5 to 1 pound of weight gain per week when an individual in outpatient treatment for an eating disorder is underweight (3).
- Severely malnourished patients must be monitored closely during nutritional rehabilitation for refeeding syndrome, which may impact the rate of weight restoration.

Weight Loss Guidelines

- No guidelines exist for recommended rate of weight loss when an eating disorder patient is overweight at the start of residential or inpatient treatment.
- Weekly or monthly weight-loss goals for overweight patients with eating disorders are not recommended because such goals heighten the focus on weight, thereby contributing to the disorder.
- Stabilization of eating behaviors takes precedence over weight loss.
- Weight maintenance without additional weight gain is an appropriate expectation during an inpatient or residential stay.
- Outpatient treatment should focus on eating behaviors that will promote weight loss over time, and encourage consistency with behaviors during periods without weight loss.

Source: Data are from reference 3.

Weight gain or loss in eating disorder recovery does not typically follow any exact pattern or maintain a constant rate over time. This unpredictability can be frustrating to patients, family members, and the treatment team, but it also offers an opportunity for nutrition education. Body weight is a consequence of eating *over time,* but many patients attempt to micromanage their weights, trying to determine which food or beverage or exact calorie amount will or did cause each weight change. Moving toward recovery requires a focus on healthy eating with little or no emphasis on minor weight fluctuations. This is a challenging change for patients to make, especially when weights are being monitored closely by the treatment team. "If my weight isn't so important, why do you have to weigh me so often?" is a common question you might hear. The appropriate answer is that the treatment team is monitoring the patient's weight so that the patient doesn't have to—so that the patient can focus on recovering a healthy relationship with food rather than trying to control his or her daily weight.

Weight changes may occasionally be dramatic, especially toward the beginning of eating disorder treatment. Patients may experience distress if they become aware of any large changes in weight. Teach patients that quick weight changes are caused by hormone fluctuations, fluid shifts, nutrient replenishment, and the movement of food and beverages through the GI tract—not by additional body mass.

When a patient expresses disappointment at a weight change or lack thereof, provide reassurance that this is a normal occurrence. Overvaluing weight as a measure of self-worth is inherent in the diagnoses of eating disorders. Failure to achieve desired weight changes therefore feels like personal failure. Act as a role model by demonstrating that weight is not relevant to your regard for your patient, and that you are proud of him or her for making the efforts that will ultimately lead to recovery. Focus on improved eating behaviors, and healthier body weight will follow. Encourage patients to refocus on eating and other actionable goals rather than using weight to measure success, and help them to look toward "a new normal" rather than "how things used to be."

Be sure to include concerned family members in your education about weight so that they bring their questions to you rather than to the patient. Teach them that weight normalization alone does not constitute a full recovery, nor is it the only indicator of recovery. Encourage patients and family members to look for other signs of progress, and to consider weight only one of many indicators.

PHYSICAL ACTIVITY

Eating disorders may involve one or more attempts to override such natural body signals as pain, injury, fatigue, and discomfort. Exercise can be used as a form of purging, a way to "earn" eating food, a mental escape from stress, a physical escape from an unhappy environment, or a pathway to admiration and a sense of accomplishment.

Patients restricted from exercise for medical reasons may become irritable and experience symptoms similar to substance withdrawal. They may choose to stand instead of sit, fidget excessively, and/or attempt to secretly exercise, even under the covers while lying in bed. Patients with severely compulsive impulses to exercise despite injuries and those who have poor bone density may need to be monitored at all times to avoid further harm.

Physical activity recommendations and/or restrictions during eating disorder treatment should be made by each patient's physician, taking into account health parameters, safety concerns, adequacy of nutrition intake, and past history of exercise compulsivity (inability to refrain from exercise even when ill, injured, or medically restricted) (4). See Box 9.2 for general guidelines. When a patient is allowed to exercise, educate him or her about the following topics:

- The energy cost of daily living, even without exercise
- The energy cost of weight restoration (for patients who are underweight), including rebuilding of bone mass, muscle mass, and organ tissue
- Physical activity as a part of healthy living, not a compensatory measure for eating
- The additional energy needs of exercise
- How to modify the meal plan to meet these additional needs

Box 9.2 General Guidelines for Physical Activity During Eating Disorder Treatment

- Recommendations for physical activity should include maximum limits for frequency, duration, and intensity (eg, "no more than 30 minutes of leisurely walking twice per week" or "no more than 45 minutes of step aerobics 3 times per week").
- Symptoms that require urgent attention (ie, chest pain, shortness of breath, muscle weakness, dizziness, heart palpitations, fatigue, heat intolerance, or other signs of distress) should be reviewed.
- Physical exercise should not be recommended for underweight patients, even when medically stable, unless they are able to meet daily energy needs plus the additional energy cost of exercise. Underweight patients may be allowed to exercise with supervision, as long as weight gain continues at an appropriate pace.
- Physical exercise should not be recommended for overweight patients, even when medically stable, if they are not eating adequate calories to meet daily energy needs.
- Patients with a history of exercise compulsivity (inability to refrain from exercise even when ill, injured, or medically restricted) or exercise as a purging method (exercising excessively in response to guilt caused by eating) should be restricted to exercising with others, in plain view of medical staff or a support person, or required to check in and out before and after exercise.

(continues next page)

Box 9.2 General Guidelines for Physical Activity During Eating Disorder Treatment (continued)

- Competitive and team sports should be discouraged until later stages of recovery. Athletes may find it difficult to respect their physical limitations and respond to signs of fatigue during competition or when others are relying on their performance.

Patients who have experienced exercise compulsivity, those who have used exercise as a purging method, and/or competitive athletes who have never experienced exercise in a leisurely manner may need to try different types of exercise to determine one or more enjoyable activities that do not trigger their eating disorder. Encourage non-competitive, social, or meditative forms of exercise, such as yoga, pilates, dance, or leisure walks.

PURGING—VOMITING, LAXATIVES, AND DIURETICS

Although self-induced vomiting, laxative abuse, and "water pills" are not effective weight-loss tools, patients report feeling "lighter," "emptier," and emotionally relieved after using these purging methods. It is important to educate patients regarding the ineffectiveness, harmful effects, and addictive nature of purging, even though education alone is not necessarily adequate to change behavior (4).

Even patients who have "quit cold turkey" from nicotine or other addictions may be surprised how difficult they find it to resist strong temptations to purge after eating. Anti-depression and/or anti-anxiety medication may be prescribed by the physician to temporarily balance brain chemistry and remove the addictive component of purging, thereby allowing behavior change techniques provided by the mental health professional to be more effective. If a patient can resist the urge to purge, it may dissipate. In addition to the guidance provided by the mental health professional, the RD may suggest additional strategies to prevent purging, such as arranging for support after meals, eating small portions frequently rather than less-frequent large meals, and abstaining from foods known to induce strong temptations to purge.

If a patient is genuinely unable to keep down any food or fluids, and/or is unable to decrease the frequency of purging behaviors, he or she should be hospitalized so that monitoring and support can be provided around the clock.

Vomiting

Chronic vomiting is damaging to teeth, gums, salivary glands, and the entire oral cavity. You can educate patients to minimize this damage after vomiting without condoning vomiting—the ultimate goal is, of course, to stop vomiting entirely.

Discourage patients from brushing their teeth immediately after vomiting, because it can further erode and damage tooth enamel beyond the effects of the stomach acid itself. Rinsing with baking soda and water will neutralize the acid and mitigate damage to the teeth. Patients whose teeth hurt when eating, drinking, or vomiting should be evaluated by a dental professional, as cavities and infection are common. An infection that enters the bloodstream or bone of the jaw can be severe.

If a patient observes blood when vomiting, insist that he or she immediately contact the physician for consultation. Blood in vomit can be a sign of broken esophageal blood vessels, or something far more serious, such as perforation of the esophageal wall. Determining a course of action in this case is not within the scope of the RD.

If a patient relates using a foreign object to induce vomiting, explain that this is a severe choking hazard. A patient who has accidentally swallowed an implement used to induce vomiting should seek emergency care in case surgical removal is required.

If a patient reports using ipecac syrup, which is used to induce vomiting in cases of accidental poison ingestion, alert the patient that ipecac builds up in the body over time and can be fatal if used repeatedly. A patient who refuses to give up using ipecac should be hospitalized.

Trigger Foods

If a patient can identify certain foods, such as "binge foods" or "trigger foods" that are known to cause inevitable urges to purge, advise him or her to avoid those foods for the time being. It is preferable for a patient to eat and keep down a nutritionally unbalanced meal rather than eating and purging one with "perfect" nutrition.

Laxatives

The assortment of available over-the-counter laxative products is astounding. Add to that the number of foods and beverages with a known or intended laxative effect, and the potential for abuse is obvious. Although laxative abuse is not an effective weight-loss tool, it does provide a "cleansing," "empty" feeling that can lead to a sense of relief after eating. Over time, a person can become psychologically and physiologically dependent on laxatives. Laxative abuse can result from a genuine need that spirals out of control. It can also develop solely as a part of the eating disorder.

There is no professional agreement on a weaning process for laxative abuse. Individuals who abuse laxatives rarely stop "cold turkey" unless they are hospitalized, and rebound constipation is possible. A GI evaluation by a physician skilled in eating disorder treatment is advised for any patient with a history of laxative abuse who reports abnormal GI function. Permanent damage to the GI tract, occasionally leading to cathartic colon and the need for surgery can occur.

In cases where a patient genuinely needs a laxative to promote normal bowel function, the physician should provide detailed guidelines for appropriate use. If the patient is not able to follow this prescription, a supportive family member or nurse (depending on the level of care) should store the medication and distribute the appropriate dose at the appropriate time. A psychiatric evaluation is also indicated due to the psychological nature of the dependence. Anti-depressant and/or anti-anxiety medication may be prescribed to allow the patient to wean successfully from laxative abuse. Behavioral interventions by the mental health professional will likely be required as well.

The RD's role in the weaning process is largely educational. Topics you may cover include the following:

- The ineffectiveness of laxatives as a weight management tool
- The potential dangers of continued use of laxatives
- The length of time that is normal for food to travel the digestive tract under natural conditions
- Recommended intakes of fluid and fiber, and types of fiber (Note: Fiber supplementation for patients with abnormal bowel function due to laxative abuse should be approved by the physician prior to recommendation by the RD.)

FOOD PROCUREMENT AND PREPARATION

Some patients with eating disorders are unequipped to independently nourish themselves. Others are very proficient in the kitchen, cooking and baking food for others while they refuse to feed themselves. For patients in the former category, your educational goals may include grocery shopping, purchasing and learning to use needed kitchen tools and supplies, learning to follow a recipe and safely use appliances, food safety and storage, and food preparation techniques. Cover these topics before you even advance to the stage of how to make an actual meal.

This introductory material may seem overly simplistic, especially if you are an accomplished cook yourself. However, keep in mind that patients with eating disorders are not functioning at their full potential. Unless they have strategies to stay safe, they could experience temptation to self-harm while using sharp knives, or fall asleep after bingeing while a pot of water boils over on the stove.

Education in situ can be especially helpful. Grocery shopping and cooking with patients, individually or in a group, can help decrease the anxiety threshold that can make these activities so intimidating. Meal management, following a recipe, drawing up a list of needed supplies—these tasks may be completely new.

Even if a patient does not wish to eat a food that you have prepared together, encounters with food (purchasing, smelling, touching, observing others eating) help build the skills needed for recovery. Discuss with a patient in advance his or her (perceived) barriers to home food preparation, and you are likely to hear anything from "I don't know what to buy," to "I don't want anyone at the grocery store to know I eat." Some barriers may not be directly related to the eating disorder. For example, a patient may have a limited food budget or have difficulty accessing places to buy food and supplies. You may need to help the patient contact a social worker who may be able to assist in finding appropriate resources, or arrange home delivery of groceries or nutritional supplements.

Every barrier has an alternative, with the one exception of "I just don't want to." If a patient is not willing to prepare his or her own food, then the timing simply is not right. There are other ways to stay nourished without having to learn to cook.

RESTAURANTS AND OTHER SOCIAL SETTINGS

Whereas some patients are unequipped to prepare their own meals and prefer eating out or "ordering in," others much prefer the comfort and control of eating only their own foods. Eating at home/in private may be effective and adequate in the early stages of recovery, but most patients will eventually need or want to eat in public—eg, at restaurants, friends' homes, or parties. Nutrition education can help them plan ahead what to eat, problem-solve tricky situations that may arise, and practice with a support person (possibly you). See Box 9.3 for possible topics.

Box 9.3 Nutrition Education Topics Related to Eating Out

- "Portion distortion" and how to manage it (eg, share an entrée, order an appetizer and a salad, put half the food in a take away container)
- Social and self-care skills (eg, asking the server to remove a complimentary bread basket or looking up a menu in advance on the Internet)
- The downside of "saving up" for one or more days in order to "splurge" during a special occasion
- Back-up strategies (eg, bringing a snack in case there is no acceptable food available when needed)
- Assertiveness when experiencing peer pressure about when, what, or where to eat

SPECIAL EVENTS

Certain situations are unpredictable and especially stressful during eating disorder recovery, even without the added stress of eating. Examples include a first date, meeting a significant other's parents, participating in a wedding, a performance, or a reunion. Help patients prepare for the eating-related aspects of these events. In addition, the mental health professional on the team can provide stress management techniques and problem-solving of social stressors that may arise.

Body image issues can flare up in advance of an event in which your patient must stand in front of a group, and the temptations of eating disorder behaviors can be strong. If patients use alcohol in social situations and/or to handle stress, take this into account. Explain that alcohol alters one's judgment regarding what and how much to eat, and help patients consider how drinking alcohol may influence their eating plan.

In extremely stressful or hostile situations, such as family gatherings where relatives are angry with the patient, you may suggest that your patient plan not to eat at the event at all, but to modify the meal plan before and after the event instead. If a patient seems unable to manage the anxiety in advance of an event with appropriate planning and problem-solving, alert the other members of the treatment team. The team may conclude that attending the event is not supportive to the patient's recovery, and a medical restriction may be the only acceptable way for the patient not to attend. If the inability to attend social or family functions is an ongoing problem, a psychiatric evaluation may be helpful in identifying a possible social anxiety disorder and corresponding treatment.

PREVENTION

Patients and their families may ask you whether eating disorders can be prevented. Current understanding of eating disorders suggests that genetic predisposition ("nature") and environmental triggers ("nurture") both play a role (5). The genetic piece cannot be prevented at this time, but the environmental dangers can potentially be reduced. Box 9.4 lists suggested methods for decreasing the environmental load that can trigger eating disorder development. Once an eating disorder has been set in motion, the most crucial dimension is obtaining care. Care should never be delayed by a parent or caregiver who fears being blamed for a child or other family member's eating disorder.

Box 9.4 Caregiver Strategies to Reduce the Risk of Eating Disorder Development

- Do not make disparaging comments on weight, body shapes, or what you or someone else is eating. Do not refer to yourself as "good" or "bad" based on what you have eaten.
- Do not keep a bathroom scale.
- Only weigh children at their medical check-ups.
- Guide children to follow their own body's signals for when, what, and how much to eat. Teach them to say "No, thanks" to food that is offered when they are not hungry.
- When a child you know is feeling down or disappointed, encourage healthful methods of expression—such as talking, writing, or art—rather than eating or dieting.
- Teach media literacy. Explain that the images we see on billboards and in print are computer-modified to appear unreal. It is not reasonable to compare our own bodies to these standards.
- When a child or teen announces a decision to change their eating, always ask why. Listen for any ulterior motive that is not food-related, such as "So I'll have more friends," or "So I'll do better in school." Teach healthful methods of handling these situations. Ask the school counselor if you are unsure what to say.
- Seek professional help for any child or teen who seems to be struggling with changes in weight, body image, or eating. If needed, seek help for yourself in order to be a better role model for healthful eating and body acceptance.

Although the degree to which societal factors actually cause eating disorders is unknown, cultural obsession with weight, fitness, dieting, and food often conceals many eating disorders until they are very severe. "Fat Talk Free Week," "Change the Message," and "Health at Every Size" are examples of awareness campaigns that spread a "body acceptance" message to combat the societal aspects of eating disorders. Spreading the word that dieting and body obsession can be harmful may contribute to the decrease of new cases of eating disorders over time.

REFERENCES

1. Tribole E. Intuitive eating in the treatment of eating disorders: the journey of attunement. *Renfrew Perspectives.* 2010;(Winter):11–14.
2. Tribole E, Resch E. *Intuitive Eating: A Revolutionary Program That Works.* 2nd ed. New York: St. Martin's Griffin; 2003.
3. Yager J, Devlin MJ, Halmi KA, Herzog DB, Mitchell JE, Powers P, Zerbe KJ. *Practice Guideline for the Treatment of Patients with Eating Disorders.* 3rd ed. Arlington, VA: American Psychiatric Association; 2006.
4. Reiter CS, Graves L. Nutrition therapy for eating disorders. *Nutr Clin Pract.* 2010;25:122–136.
5. American Dietetic Association. Position of the American Dietetic Association: nutrition intervention in the treatment of anorexia nervosa, bulimia nervosa, and other eating disorders. *J Am Diet Assoc.* 2006;106:2073–2082.

Chapter 10

Nutrition Counseling Interventions

INTRODUCTION

Nutrition counseling for eating disorders is "eclectic," meaning that the registered dietitian (RD) can choose from among a variety of counseling techniques depending on each patient's needs. This chapter describes some of the counseling tools commonly used to treat eating disorders and addresses some of the challenges facing the RD during the nutrition counseling process. The chapter concludes with guidelines for the duration of nutrition counseling for eating disorders and additional counseling resources.

MOTIVATIONAL INTERVIEWING AND READINESS FOR CHANGE

For many nutrition counseling interventions, success relies heavily on the patient's willingness to work toward recovery, confidence that change is achievable, and ability to persevere in the face of inevitable difficulties. In the transtheoretical model, this is described as "readiness for change" (1).

Motivational interviewing (MI) is a counseling technique to assess the patient's level of motivation to change and help him or her shift from precontemplative, contemplative, and preparation stages into action (2). MI techniques include active and reflective listening, open-ended questions, affirmation, and summarization, all of which are appropriate in nutrition counseling (3).

Even when progress seems to stagnate or slow down, or when patients express a desire to change that is unmatched by action ("resistance to change"), patients can benefit from encouragement to find their own motivation to change. It increases their investment in recovery and therefore helps prevent relapse.

Patients who are so malnourished or mentally unwell that they cannot think rationally are not appropriate candidates for MI by the RD. Patients who are hospitalized against their will because their refusal to change puts their life in danger are also unsuited for MI. As long they remain medically stable, the remaining majority of patients in treatment for eating disorders can benefit from nutrition counseling using MI.

Patients who are simultaneously motivated and reluctant to change are prime candidates for MI. The RD can use MI to explore this ambivalence on the surface level of food and eating behaviors. However, fear of failure and other emotional issues must be addressed by a mental health professional. Patients may wish to focus solely on food interventions, as they can distract from more painful psychological issues, but this narrow focus prevents true recovery. In these situations, consult with other treatment team members, a trusted colleague, or a supervisor to help you evaluate whether to "push" the patient to attempt eating interventions or to support the patient in maintaining the status quo until barriers to action have been addressed in therapy. Explain to the patient and family that conscious motivation and desire are not the only factors in eating disorder recovery, just as weight restoration and balanced eating are not the only goals.

Using MI, the RD and the patient share the responsibility of evaluating the patient's readiness for new interventions. The following example demonstrates this process:

- The RD suggests that the patient make a change on an experimental basis (eg, to refrain from weighing for 24 hours), as a way of gathering information about readiness.
- The RD and patient discuss the results of the experiment (the patient refrained from weighing but did not eat during the 24-hour period) to determine whether the new behavior can be adopted on a more regular basis. In this case, the negative repercussions indicate that changing this particular behavior is not supportive to the patient's recovery at this time.
- Before attempting the behavior again, the RD and patient identify alternate possibilities to obtain the same result (eg, the RD will weigh the patient backward so that the weight is monitored but the patient does not see it), along with other factors that could make the new behavior more successful (eg, the 24 hours without weighing will be the day immediately preceding the next session with the RD).

In this way, the RD not only provides helpful recommendations for the patient but also serves as a role model for several qualities important to eating disorder recovery: (*a*) the ability to attempt an intervention without guarantee of a perfect outcome, (*b*) acceptance without self-blame when expectations are not met; and (*c*) a willingness to try again. These are important "coping skills" that help patients tolerate and/or counteract the feelings of guilt, wrongdoing, and shame that often result from the changes necessary to recovery.

COPING SKILLS

Coping skills are the tools that patients require to change their eating patterns from disordered to healthy. Eating disorder behaviors persist beyond reason because they seem to "work." Therefore, patients who wish to discard these behaviors need to learn alternate skills with comparable results. MI is the first step; developing coping skills is the next.

Many eating disorder behaviors require coping skills for both nutrition-related and psychological aspects. The RD should assist with the nutrition issues and the mental health counselor with the others. For example, if a patient binge eats every evening in lieu of dinner, the RD and patient will attempt to discern the rationale behind the binge eating and the skills necessary to replace it.

If the binge eating is related to coming home ravenous after work, inadequate planning for the evening meal, inability to cook or grocery shop, or fear of weight gain from eating after a certain hour, the RD can teach coping skills for these problems. They may include skills for eating during the day to avoid coming home ravenous, preparing an evening meal after a busy work day, making a menu and grocery shopping for the week, managing unrealistic fears of weight gain, and so on.

If the binge eating behavior is also driven by work stress, feelings of inadequacy, a desire to escape from the responsibilities of family life, or other non-nutrition related issues, the mental health counselor will be needed to assist the patient with strategies for managing these factors.

Additional coping skills will be necessary as nutrition interventions progress, higher calorie foods are introduced, weight changes accumulate, and the level of care changes (4). Challenges of recovery itself include peer reactions to changes in body size, fear of failure to maintain recovery, and realization that recovery is a long-term process. Coping skills are therefore needed for managing the stress of recovery itself.

Strategies that RDs can use to help patients cope include the following:

- Planning ahead for eating situations, such as looking up restaurant menus online
- Problem solving possible solutions for difficult situations that may arise
- Role-playing imaginary situations that may trigger behavior or feelings
- Devising a list of supportive activities and people to distract from stressful feelings after eating
- "Legalizing" food and other types of nutrition education (see Chapter 9)
- Writing a log of thoughts and feelings before and/or after eating
- Creating notes with helpful information and reminders to be reviewed before and/or after eating

The RD can assist the patient both with *external* strategies (eg, stay out of the bathroom for 1 hour after meals) and *internal* strategies (eg, remind yourself that you know people who eat cream cheese and are not overweight). During the initial stages of treatment, coping strategies are usually externally based, with internal structure developing over time.

COGNITIVE BEHAVIORAL THERAPY

Cognitive behavioral therapy (CBT) is based on the concept that behaviors are caused by feelings and that feelings are caused by thoughts. It is the most thoroughly studied counseling technique in nutrition therapy and the treatment of eating disorders (3), and can be used together with MI.

The purpose of CBT in eating disorder treatment is to help patients recognize that eating disorder behaviors are caused by *thoughts* about food, not by the foods themselves. CBT is therefore a perfect fit with the concept of legalizing food and removing "good" vs "bad" labels (see Chapter 9). To improve behaviors, first change the thoughts associated with them.

CBT requires time, attention, and willingness to change. Therefore, it is not an appropriate strategy for extremely malnourished, mentally unwell, defiant, or medically unstable patients. Once these patients have been nutritionally restored and physically and mentally stabilized, they may attempt CBT for continued recovery.

Other candidates for nutrition counseling with CBT are patients who no longer actively practice eating disorder behaviors but are still consumed with thoughts and fears about food. These patients have improved eating behaviors, but they have not truly recovered until they change the internal eating disorder environment (5).

When patients agree to a nutrition intervention that challenges the eating disorder (eg, eating more calories; a social eating situation; a food challenge), they can usually expect to feel an emotional backlash. Using CBT, the RD can help the patient plan ahead for how to manage uncomfortable thoughts and feelings that arise before or after the challenge, such as "I can't eat pizza without purging," "I'm going to get fat if I don't know how many calories are in that meal," or "If people see me eat, they will think I'm disgusting."

CBT provides a format for addressing these negative thoughts and feelings based on its foundational premise that these feelings are not related to the events, but to the individual patient's own beliefs. In the first example, "I ate pizza; I need to get rid of it," the RD can use CBT principles to show the patient that pizza is an inanimate object, incapable of causing feelings. Therefore, eating pizza does not cause the desire to purge. The desire to purge stems from the patient's internal beliefs about pizza. The simple question, "What is it that you believe about pizza that makes it so bad?" can present opportunities for appropriate nutrition education. Perhaps the patient holds a mistaken belief that pizza causes weight gain. This mistaken *belief* (and not the *behavior* of eating pizza) is what causes the guilt/fear/feeling of wrongdoing that leads to purging.

Patients may struggle to grasp these sorts of distinctions—"Pizza must be purged!" seems so true and real, whereas "Pizza is a safe food; I can eat pizza without gaining weight" seems so unbelievable. CBT provides a framework to combine nutrition education (the facts) with nutrition counseling (overcoming barriers to change), while recognizing that a change in thinking is progress even before it leads to a change in behavior. Perhaps the patient in this example reports that the following week she was presented with the option of eating pizza. She chose not to eat it. However, this time she made her choice based on the facts ("I am scared of eating pizza because for a long time I told myself it would make me fat"), rather than on the eating disorder myth ("Pizza will make me fat"). Although the patient did not eat pizza, she also did not restrict and eat nothing, nor did she eat pizza and purge. The door is opened for the patient to eat pizza in the future and, more importantly, for her to change even more negative thoughts about food over time.

In the future, the RD may teach the patient how to incorporate pizza into a healthy meal plan, or encourage the patient to accept the challenge experiment of eating a piece of pizza. The RD can assist the patient in developing coping skills in preparation for the negative feelings that may result. The short-term goal is for the patient to separate pizza from her thoughts about pizza. The intermediate goal is for her to eat a piece of pizza and successfully handle the guilty feelings associated with this action. The long-term goal is for her to detach almost entirely her feelings of guilt from the experience of food.

Clearly, change with CBT is a slow and painstaking process. Each patient has many thoughts and feelings that drive the eating disorder cycle. Once again, the RD has the opportunity to model coping skills, such as patience; managing frustration without placing blame or quitting; and identifying progress when it is not obvious.

ESTABLISHING HEALTHY BOUNDARIES IN NUTRITION COUNSELING

RDs who do not have additional mental health credentials should limit nutrition counseling to objectives within the RD's scope of practice. The following strategies are suggested and discussed here:

- Focus sessions primarily on nutrition
- Make appropriate referrals
- Reinforce the team approach to treatment
- Address boundary violations

Focus Sessions Primarily on Nutrition

As you develop a good working relationship with a patient, you may find that conversations flow toward and then away from nutrition-related topics. Striking the right balance between nutrition counseling and chit-chat is essential, but it takes time. Remember that for most eating disorder patients, you are one of only a few people who have access to very personal information. Therefore, your patients may need time to transition from small talk to serious business when they come in from the "outside world." If small talk or "How was your week?" responses start to take up too much of your allotted time, use a transitional statement to move to the topic of nutrition. (See Box 10.1.) If your attempts at making gentle transitions are ineffective, try saying, "I've enjoyed hearing about that" or "I'm sorry to hear about that." Continue with, "I would like to hear more, but I'm concerned that we won't have time left for what we need to cover. Can we switch over to nutrition and your meal plan?"

Box 10.1 Examples of Transitional Statements

- "That's so interesting! I'm curious how that affected your eating."
- "Oh, that's a bummer! I wonder how that might have turned out differently if you didn't have an eating disorder?"
- "I'm so glad you had that experience! Tell me—did it make a difference in your eating?"
- "That does sound like a great weekend! Do you think your eating disorder played a role in how it turned out?"

Make Appropriate Referrals to Mental Health Counseling

The separation of eating from unrelated emotions is an ongoing process in eating disorder recovery. As a facilitator of this recovery, you may wonder at times whether you are leaving the scope of practice of an RD and crossing into the "territory" of the mental health professional (6,7). Monitoring the distinction between your role and that of a mental health counselor is a healthy sign of self-awareness and reflective of your desire to practice in an ethical manner. Although the dividing line may sometimes seem blurry, there is a distinct category of topics that falls within the scope of the RD: anything that relates to or influences food and/or eating (8). As long as assessment, education, and interventions with your patients revolve around and relate to these topics, you are working within your scope.

When topics that seem unrelated to food and eating arise during nutrition counseling, as they often do, guide the conversation to food with a question, such as: "How do you think that affected your eating?" Many situations that are not about food on the surface have some connection to nutrition or eating, especially for an individual working to heal from an eating disorder.

When a patient brings to your attention a concern or event unrelated to food, eating or nutrition, you can remain within the RD's scope of practice by recommending that the patient discuss this topic with his or her counselor. Listening to your patient's non-nutrition concerns does not take you out of the RD's scope of practice. In fact, consider your patient's trust in you to be a compliment. Then use your response, such as, "That is an important topic to discuss with your counselor" to validate the significance of the issue while guiding the patient to the more appropriate treatment provider.

See Box 10.2 and Chapter 11 for guidance on referring patients who do not have already have a counselor.

Box 10.2 Referrals to Counselors

Many patients with eating disorders seek the services of a registered dietitian because they think that their issues are solely rooted in nutrition and can be solved with nutrition intervention alone. Whether they simply are unaware of the help a mental health professional can provide, or they are resistant to obtaining this type of help, the RD can offer a sensitive and caring referral. A simple way to phrase this recommendation is, "I can see that this is an important area for you to discuss, but I know I'm not the best person to advise you on that. Have you ever considered meeting with a counselor?"

If you are not familiar with the counselors in your area who are experienced with eating disorder work, you can always suggest that patients ask their physician for a recommendation. See Chapter 11 for more information about referring a patient to other forms of therapy.

Reinforce the Team Approach to Treatment

Because of the RD's role as a supportive member of the treatment team, patients and family members may ask you for general guidance unrelated to nutrition. In most cases, you should direct these questions to a physician or therapist, rather than answering directly. Such questions can seem like simple requests for your opinion ("Do you think our daughter will be ready to go to college in the fall?"). However, they are usually more complex and require thorough discussion. In some circumstances, they may even be manipulative attempts to pit members of the treatment team against each other ("splitting"), and you may be unhappily surprised to hear your words used against you later.

Even under ideal circumstances, in which your patients and their family members do not seek your advice casually, you should keep in mind that they will view any opinions you share as authoritative because you are a member of the treatment team. Therefore, you should discuss any requests to make changes to the treatment plan with other team members before offering a definitive decision to patient or family.

At the same time, you must remember that the patient and family are in crisis and may not be hearing or interpreting information well or accurately. Whenever a patient or family member repeats something another provider said or did that sounds irregular, consider double-checking the situation with the other provider. These checks are especially helpful when a patient or family member criticizes another provider or indicates that another provider criticized you. These kinds of comments are not always conscious efforts to disrupt treatment, but they certainly do.

Just as eating disorders can twist how individuals think about food, leading them to categorize each food and each eating episode as "all good" or "all bad," patients may think of people in absolute terms. An individual in treatment for an eating disorder may "warm up" to one member of the treatment team more so than the others. If you are this chosen ally, proceed with caution.

You may feel satisfied, or even proud, if a generally grumpy patient cheers up when you enter the room. Just remember that everything is not as simple as it seems. The same patient who thinks you are great when you change her meal plan today may express anger when you change it back tomorrow. You cannot let the patient manipulate you by giving you the cold shoulder or granting you special favors. Most of all, do not believe at face value any patient's assertions that another treatment team member is unfair, difficult, or incorrect. Encourage the patient to bring such concerns to the person in question.

Otherwise, you assist the patient in subverting his or her own recovery. If a patient gives you information from another treatment provider that sounds questionable, always take the time to verify the information directly with the other professional.

Address Boundary Violations

At times, you may be tempted to relate personally to a patient in your care, especially if he or she is close to you in age, reminds you of someone you know, grew up in your hometown, or shares other characteristics with you. Perhaps you imagine that the two of you would have become friends under different circumstances. However, your relationship as RD and patient cannot move past certain professional boundaries.

Patients can unconsciously diminish the authority of their providers by treating them like peers or friends. Bringing you a coffee, offering to fix you up on a date, calling you by a nickname—all of these are examples of simple ways that a patient may attempt to decrease the power differential between the two of you. In these situations, speak with another provider on the team (especially a mental health provider) to gauge the significance of this behavior and the potential harm or benefits of discussing it with the patient.

In some cases, you may decide to "leave it alone" and not mention the attempted boundary violations to the patient, while consciously keeping your boundaries and actions professional. In other cases, with the support of your treatment team, you or the therapist may comment to the patient on his or her behavior and express your wishes that your relationship stay strictly professional.

When patients are learning new ways of behaving, as they must to recover, receiving redirection from you or another member of the treatment team can feel like a rejection that then impairs your working relationship. Nevertheless, you should not remain in uncomfortable situations to avoid "rocking the boat" with a patient. Speaking with another professional (even one who does not know the patient, as in professional supervision or mentoring) is the best way to determine your course of action, whether verbal redirection, intervention from another member of the treatment team or a supervisor, or other options.

If a patient fails to attend scheduled appointments, does not pay you the agreed-upon fee, is not compliant with recommendations that you think are essential for the patient's safety, or is threatening to you or your staff, you should definitely tell the patient that you will not continue to be part of the treatment team unless certain conditions (which you specify) are met. Such conversations can feel confrontational and even emotional, so keep in mind that setting these boundaries is an intervention in the best interest of the patient, and once again seek support from the team, a colleague or your supervisor.

COUNSELING STRATEGIES FOR TIMES WHEN PATIENTS ARE VERY EMOTIONAL

You may occasionally meet with a patient who is experiencing very strong feelings. These feelings may or may not be eating disorder–related. If they are related ("I'm devastated that I can't go to college because of my eating disorder!"), you may be able to use a transitional statement or channel the conversation toward what can be done to advance recovery. Try to validate the patient's feelings first, and then transition. In response to the patient who cannot attend college, you might say, "I can see that you're really disappointed and that you want to go to college. Let's look at what needs to happen with your eating so that you can go another semester."

Other strong feelings your patients may express are not related in any way to the eating disorder, but are simply overpowering ("My grandfather died. I leave tomorrow for his funeral. I am devastated!"). These feelings defy any transitional statement or segue to nutrition. You are left with two options to offer the patient—always remembering to validate!—"That's awful! I'm so sorry to hear about your grandfather. Do you want to have a session with me, or would your time be better used getting ready for your trip?"

Support your patient on whichever choice he or she makes. If you sense that your patient is trying to please you by staying when he or she really wants or needs to leave, you may "pull rank" and say, "I can tell you are tempted to stay, but that you really want [or need] to leave. I support you in leaving. It won't hurt my feelings, and we can pick up where we left off when you come back."

It is always wise to convey some information to the other treatment team members about a patient's strong feelings. Share your knowledge of the situation and your decision to end your session early or continue it.

COUNSELING STRATEGIES TO ADDRESS PATIENT ANGER OR HOSTILITY

When patients express anger regarding the process of treatment or recovery, encourage them to share their feelings with the mental health professional on the team. Remain neutral or express your understanding that anger is an expected emotion during the recovery process. If a patient inappropriately directs anger at you, follow your facility protocol, or leave the room, explaining that you are giving the patient an opportunity to calm down. If a patient becomes threatening or violent, call security or follow the facility protocol. Report the patient's behavior and your response to the other members of the treatment team.

If anger at the slow pace of recovery turns to hopelessness, and the patient indicates a wish to die, give up, or not be alive, this should be immediately reported to the mental health professional or physician who can evaluate whether hospitalization is necessary.

Hostile behavior may be a defense mechanism or a symptom of a personality disorder, substance abuse, or other mental illness. Report the patient's behavior to your supervisor and the other members of the treatment team. Ask for advice on whether to continue to approach the patient, or whether it is more appropriate to work behind the scenes until the patient is more approachable.

COUNSELING PATIENTS WITH PERSONALITY DISORDERS

Personality disorders can occur concurrently with eating disorders, but they are not diagnosed as easily because the behaviors are not always apparent (9). When a patient in your care is diagnosed with a personality disorder, ask for guidance from the other members of the team. Of course, an RD cannot treat the patient for the personality disorder, but your nutrition counseling may be influenced by the patient's particular personality traits, as the following examples illustrate:

- An eating disorder patient with narcissistic personality disorder seems disgruntled when you make suggestions about his eating, even though you both are aware that that is your job. The next time you meet, he reports doing exactly what you suggested but describes his actions as if they were his original idea. Express your frustration with your support system rather than the patient, and be proud that you helped the patient to a positive outcome, even if you do not get the credit.
- An eating disorder patient with borderline personality disorder acts as if she will never survive if you meet only twice per week, instead of every day—you are her lifeline! Then, instead of coming back for the next appointment, she finds a new RD, essentially leaving you before you could "abandon" her. You are unlikely to resolve this situation with the patient. Discuss your feelings with your own supportive resources, and recognize that you did not do anything wrong.

Intentionally or unintentionally, individuals with personality disorders are very good at making others feel badly. Professional supervision will assist you in accepting the feelings and reactions ("countertransference") you may experience. For more information about personality disorders, refer to the resources noted in Box 10.3.

Box 10.3 Further Reading About Personality Disorders

Hotchkiss S. *Why Is It Always About You? The Seven Deadly Sins of Narcissism*. New York, NY: Free Press; 2003.
Kreisman JJ. *I Hate You, Don't Leave Me: Understanding the Borderline Personality*. New York, NY: Avon Books; 1989.
Lawson CA. *Understanding the Borderline Mother: Helping Her Children Transcend the Intense, Unpredictable, and Volatile Relationship*. Lanham, MD: Jason Aronson; 2002.
Payson ED. *The Wizard of Oz and Other Narcissists: Coping with the One-Way Relationship in Work, Love, and Family*. Royal Oak, MI: Julian Day Publications; 2002.
Sansone RA, Levitt JL, ed. *Personality Disorders and Eating Disorders: Exploring the Frontier*. New York, NY: Taylor and Francis; 2006.

COUNSELING STRATEGIES TO ADDRESS DEFENSE MECHANISMS

Coping skills are conscious, healthy tools for becoming aware of and handling distressing feelings. Defense mechanisms are the opposite—unconscious, potentially unhealthy methods for avoiding these feelings altogether. Box 10.4 (10,11) lists the defense mechanisms that often are linked to eating disorders.

Box 10.4 Defense Mechanisms Related to Eating Disorders

- **Altruism**: Helping others. This becomes a defense when it is used to avoid unwanted feelings or foods. *Example*: "I couldn't follow my meal plan because I spent all day at the animal shelter."
- **Asceticism**: The renunciation of certain pleasures to avoid the anxiety and conflict associated with them. *Example*: "I don't like ice cream, it's too rich. I like my food very plain."

(continues next page)

Box 10.4 Defense Mechanisms Related to Eating Disorders (continued)

- **Compensation**: Trying to make up for perceived deficiencies. *Example*: "They may ignore me at the party, but at least I will be the skinniest person there."
- **Denial**: A direct negation or refusal to accept painful or unwanted aspects of reality. (A certain amount of denial allows us to function in the world, but it becomes problematic when it distorts reality.) *Example*: "I could stop my eating disorder any time if I wanted to."
- **Intellectualization**: Thinking and talking about feelings and impulses rather than feeling them. *Example*: "I don't eat because I just never feel hungry. I watch cooking shows all day but it's not because I have an eating disorder. I just really like them. "
- **Projection**: Attributing unwanted thoughts and feelings to others. *Example*: "I didn't follow my meal plan this week. I know you're so disappointed in me."
- **Regression**: The return to an earlier developmental stage or type of behavior to avoid present anxiety. *Example*: "I know I was eating higher-fat foods last week, but this week I have so much going on, I just can't deal with all that fat."
- **Repression**: Keeping unwanted thoughts or feelings completely out of awareness. *Example*: "No, I've never been unhappy before now. If I didn't have this eating disorder, I'd be stress-free!"
- **Somatization**: Converting intolerable conflict into physical symptoms. *Example*: "I can't increase my calories. I get immediate migraines if I eat more than this many calories a day."
- **Splitting:** Categorizing people, things, and time periods as either "all good" or "all bad" (also known as "black-and-white thinking"). *Example*: "Once I eat a cookie, I might as well have a binge. I mean it's already a bad day, so why not go all out."

Source: Data are from references 10 and 11.

Defense mechanisms become a problem when they interfere with reality or interpersonal relations. In some cases, a patient's unconscious defense mechanisms may be irrelevant to the RD's counseling strategies. In others, the defense mechanisms may directly impair a patient's efforts to change, or willingness to participate in nutrition counseling at all.

A lack of cooperation (eg, refusal to complete assignments; refusal to attend or speak during nutrition counseling sessions; and/or insistence that nutrition counseling is unnecessary) can be a passive-aggressive defense mechanism to conceal feelings of inadequacy or fear of abandonment. It is important to not take this behavior personally and to communicate with other members of the treatment team who can provide guidance (to you) and/or consequences (to the patient). Your calm, nonjudgmental responses and willingness to work with the patient may slowly generate the rapport necessary to move forward in nutrition counseling.

Discuss your observations of all defensive behavior with the mental health professional on the treatment team. He or she may be able to address the defenses with the patient and/or suggest strategies that you can use.

If a medically unstable patient minimizes or denies the severity of illness, consult the patient's physician about whether it is safe for you to continue meeting with the patient. If the patient does not have a physician, consult your supervisor.

ADDRESSING HOPELESSNESS

Eating disorders often co-occur with depression, which may be pre-existing or caused by the eating disorder. The following strategies are suggested for RDs working with patients that exhibit signs of hopelessness or severe depression:

- A peer support group or online mentor may be helpful in providing a message of hope that recovery is indeed possible.
- If the patient has not been treated for depression, refer him or her for psychiatric evaluation. Severe depression can lead to hopelessness or thoughts of suicide, in addition to a lack of interest in food. Malnutrition can decrease the efficacy of some antidepressant medications, creating a downward spiral that is difficult to break on an outpatient basis. A higher level of care may be necessary to ensure the patient's safety and stabilize the depression.
- When you suspect that depression is impairing a patient's willingness to change, capacity to believe that change is even possible, and/or ability to make use of nutrition counseling sessions, speak with other members of the treatment team for guidance.
- If a patient expresses hopelessness or thoughts of suicide and you are concerned about his or her safety, contact one of the mental health professionals on the team *immediately* for guidance. If you are unable to reach another team member, call the patient's emergency contact and ask this person to stay with the patient until a mental health professional is available.

DURATION OF NUTRITION COUNSELING

No consensus exists for the expected duration of eating disorder treatment or nutrition counseling for eating disorders. True recovery is a long-term, perhaps lifelong, process. Unrealistic expectations for the pace of recovery can manifest in frustration at the slow pace of progress and even anger at the RD and other members of the treatment team.

Some patients start to regress as they draw close to the end of treatment and the day when they can finally consider themselves "recovered." There are many reasons why this occurs—patients may have expected that recovery "would be different," that they would be happier or treated differently by others; recovery may be linked with a fearful transition, such as leaving for college or becoming a parent; or certain issues may not be recognized for their significance until treatment appears nearly complete, and patients realize they will soon be meeting the challenges of life without the structure provided by treatment team.

For these reasons, nutrition counseling should not be terminated when a patient reaches a certain weight goal, discharge date, or intake level. When discharged from inpatient or residential treatment, patients should be provided with contact information for an outpatient RD in the area in which they live.

As a patient becomes able to handle eating challenges with less-frequent intervention from the RD, nutrition counseling should be gradually decreased in frequency, but it should not be stopped completely until the patient has experienced at least 6 months of remission. Nutrition counseling ultimately should continue on an as-needed basis. It should not have a "termination" or "graduation" date after which the patient may not contact the RD.

Throughout their lives, patients continue to experience new challenges in life, both positive and negative, therefore recovery and maintaining appropriate eating may be challenged as well. When transitioning from regularly scheduled visits with the RD to an as-needed basis, the RD and patient should review criteria for making an appointment. Criteria should be specific to the patient and should include indications that the patient is struggling (eg, a weight change [increase or decrease] of a specified number of pounds, or increasing thoughts and fears about eating) as well as life changes that would require a change in eating schedule or nutrition needs (eg a new job, becoming pregnant).

Some patients may express concerns that continuing to meet with the RD is a sign of weakness or failure in recovery. Encourage them to regard reaching out to the RD for help when needed as a positive coping skill.

EXPANDING YOUR NUTRITION COUNSELING SKILLS

RDs who continue to learn about eating disorders, counseling techniques, and psychotherapy, will encounter many therapeutic tools and theories (see Box 10.5). RDs do not practice all of these therapies—in many cases, they require special training, credentials, and equipment. However, as an "eclectic" form of therapy, nutrition counseling can pull from a variety of sources to facilitate behavior change and healing (8,10,11).

Box 10.5 Selected Therapies Used in Eating Disorder Treatment

- Rational emotive behavior theory
- Emotion acceptance behavior therapy
- Acceptance and commitment therapy
- Dialectical behavioral therapy
- Cognitive remediation therapy
- Family systems theory
- Psychodrama
- Eye movement desensitization therapy
- Bio- and neurofeedback
- Exposure therapy
- Integrative cognitive affective therapy
- Equine-assisted therapy
- Expressive therapy (art, drama, music, dance)

If you are interested in learning more about the counseling theories described in this chapter, refer to the resources listed in Box 10.6. Refer also to Appendix C, which identifies additional books and resources by RDs to help with counseling skills for eating disorders.

Box 10.6 Further Reading on Counseling Theories

Arkowitz H, Miller W, Rollnick S, Westra H. *Motivational Interviewing in the Treatment of Psychological Problems.* New York, NY: Guilford Press; 2008._

Beck AT. *Cognitive Therapy and the Emotional Disorders.* New York, NY: Penguin; 1979.

Fairburn CG. *Cognitive Behavioral Therapy and Eating Disorders.* New York, NY: Guilford Press; 2008.

Natenshon A. *Doing What Works: An Integrative System for Treating Eating Disorders from Diagnosis to Recovery.* Washington, DC: NASW Press; 2009.

Safer D, Telch C, Chen E, Linehan M. *Dialectical Behavior Therapy for Binge Eating and Bulimia.* New York, NY: Guilford Press; 2009.

REFERENCES

1. Prochaska JO, Norcross JC, DiClemente V. *Changing for Good: A Revolutionary Six-Stage Program for Overcoming Bad Habits and Moving Your Life Positively Forward.* New York, NY: Avon Books; 1994.
2. Bewell-Weiss C, Carter J. Motivational interviewing in the treatment of eating disorders. *Renfrew Perspect.* 2010;(Winter):4–6.
3. Spahn JM, Reeves RS, Keim KS, LaQuatra I, Kellogg M, Jortberg B, Clark NA. State of the evidence regarding behavior change strategies in nutrition counseling to facilitate health and food behavior change. *J Am Diet Assoc.* 2010;110:879–891.
4. Kleifield EI, Wagner S, Halmi KA. Cognitive-behavioral treatment of anorexia nervosa. *Psych Clin N Am.* 1996;19:715–737.
5. Crow S. Recovery from eating disorders. *Renfrew Perspect.* 2007;(Winter):1–3.
6. Salloff-Coste C, Hamburg P, Herzog D. Nutrition and psychotherapy: collaborative treatment of patients with eating disorders. *Bull Menninger Clin.* 1993;57:504–516.
7. Kellogg M. When and how to refer to psychotherapy. *Weight Management Matters.* 2008;6(2):14–15.
8. Reiter CS, Graves L. Nutrition therapy for eating disorders. *Nutr Clin Pract.* 2010;25:122–136.
9. Sansone RA, Levitt JL, eds. *Personality Disorders and Eating Disorders: Exploring the Frontier.* New York, NY: Routledge; 2006.
10. Negri M, Setnick J. What's eating your patients? Solving emotional eating from the inside out. *Bariatric Times.* 2006;3(1).
11. Kratina K, King NL, Hayes D. *Moving Away from Diets: Healing Eating Problems and Exercise Resistance.* 2nd ed. Denton, TX: Helm Publishing; 2003.

Chapter 11

Coordination of Care Nutrition Interventions

INTRODUCTION

At its most basic, eating disorder treatment involves a physician and/or psychiatrist, a registered dietitian (RD), and a mental health professional. This chapter addresses topics related to the coordination of care between the RD and other members of the treatment team and concludes with a brief discussion of reimbursement issues.

COMMUNICATING WITH OTHER PROVIDERS

During or prior to your initial nutrition assessment of the patient, obtain permission to communicate with other treatment providers (including providers you recommend). If you work in a facility, this permission may be handled on behalf of all providers at the time of admission. If you work independently, you will need to gather permission releases along with names and contact information. Together with the patient and the patient's family members, these providers and you comprise the treatment team. All members of the team should be included in major treatment decisions.

After completing your initial nutrition assessment, follow up with each of the other treatment team members (either in person or by e-mail, fax, or phone call) to obtain additional information and provide a summary of your assessment and recommendations. If you work in a facility, "case conferences," rounds, or treatment team meetings are ideal times to share information and confer about treatment plans.

If you work independently, you may need to first assist your patient in locating other providers. Once the treatment team is selected, you and the other providers can agree on preferred methods of conveying and receiving information. At the beginning of treatment, communication may be very frequent. As the patient progresses into recovery, communication may proceed on as "as needed" basis (ie, communication only when treatment changes or problems develop) or at regular intervals (eg, weekly, monthly, or every visit).

WORKING WITH MENTAL HEALTH CARE PROFESSIONALS

Mental health care includes both psychotherapy ("counseling") and psychiatry, two important and often essential modalities in the treatment of eating disorders (1). Psychotherapy can take many forms and is provided by a variety of practitioners. Learn the credentials for licensed mental health providers in your state. These may include psychologists, nurses, nurse practitioners, social workers, licensed professional counselors, guidance counselors, family therapists, analysts, youth pastors, ministers, rabbis, chaplains, and others. Depending on each patient's diagnosis and needs, different types of counselors and counseling may be appropriate.

It is helpful when the counselor has some familiarity with eating disorder treatment theories, even if he or she is not exclusively an eating disorder specialist. Some counselors use eclectic techniques, similar to those of

RDs; others specialize in cognitive behavioral therapy, dialectical behavioral therapy, or other methods helpful in eating disorder recovery. The ideal counselor offers evidence-based treatment and is a good personality match with the patient. To find a successful match, a patient may choose to meet with more than one counselor. Box 11.1 summarizes specific situations and topics that can be addressed with psychotherapy.

Box 11.1 Reasons to Refer Patients to a Mental Health Professional

- Diagnosis of psychiatric illness, including an eating disorder
- Relationship or family problems, recent or past
- Difficulty adjusting to a recent life change
- Behavior changes as a result of stress or life events
- Difficulty caring for self or children, difficulty with activities of daily living
- Traumatic event(s), including diagnosis of severe, stigmatizing, or debilitating illness and medical recommendations that change quality of life (eg, bed rest, chemotherapy, insulin shots)
- Depression, anxiety, or other overwhelming emotions, whether reported or observed (crying in session, agitation, pacing, anger, etc)
- Family member(s) are preoccupied with patient's weight or eating
- Sudden change in behavior, mood, or mental state, reported or observed
- Inability to change even though expressing desire to change
- Fears, anxiety, or stress (whether warranted or unwarranted) about the course of the eating disorder or recovery

You may encounter patients who disagree with or disapprove of your recommendation that they pursue counseling. Other patients may tell you that they "have already done that" and are not willing to "do it again." Box 11.2 lists suggested ways to encourage your patients to seek mental health care.

Box 11.2 Overcoming Patient Objections to Mental Health Care

- Explain your rationale for your recommendation that the patient seek care. Specify which issues you are recommending for counseling, rather than making a general recommendation for "therapy" or "counseling." For example, to a patient who is overwhelmed with commitments, explain "I think this counselor could really help you with time management."
- Listen to the patient's point of view and respond to his or her concerns. If the patient is concerned about something specific, you may be able to address those fears directly. For example, you might respond, "I understand that you didn't have a good experience with a previous counselor. You certainly don't have to go back to that person. There are many other options that I can suggest, if you'd like," or "I understand that you don't want to talk about your childhood experiences. That would be a great thing to tell a counselor, as well as the things you *do* want to work on."
- Encourage patients to consider an evaluation of a new therapist as an interview, and to try more than one therapist if that helps them find a good match.
- To a patient who says, "But I really like talking with you. I don't understand why you want me to see someone else," respond with, "I agree we've done a lot together, and I'm glad that you feel comfortable talking with me. However, in this case, I'm not the best person to give you advice. I'd like to help you find a counselor with whom you feel just as comfortable."

(continues next page)

Box 11.2 Overcoming Patient Objections to Mental Health Care (continued)

- To a patient who does not understand how a counselor can help, you might say, "We have been working together for a while on this issue, and in my experience, when someone wants to change and can't, there is often something behind it. A counselor is the type of person who can help you find that stumbling block so that our work together will succeed."
- To a patient who resists seeing a counselor because "things are going fine right now," suggest one visit, just as a backup plan—"Things are going great now, and I'm glad. However, I'm concerned that eventually life might present more challenges again. So right now, while life is nice and calm, check out a couple of therapists and see who you like. Just go once or twice to get to know them a little. That way if a crisis hits, we'll be prepared."
- When a patient adamantly refuses to agree to try a counselor, you have three options:
  - Keep a running list of topics you think the patient could address in counseling. Keep this list with your patient's chart and inform the patient each time you add a topic. Your actions will show the patient three things: (*a*) these are the type of topics appropriate for counseling; (*b*) you do not intend to discuss these topics; and (*c*) there really are issues to discuss with a counselor. It is up to you how long you keep this up until you move to the next step.
  - Set a time limit. For example, tell the patient, "I understand you are hesitant about seeing a counselor and you feel that my help is enough to get through this problem. Let's make a deal. Let's give ourselves 3 weeks to keep at it. Then we'll reevaluate your situation. If things aren't better, you will agree to meet up with a counselor." If at the appointed time your patient still refuses, you are left with the last resort.

(continues next page)

Box 11.2 Overcoming Patient Objections to Mental Health Care (continued)

- ◦ Refuse to contine nutrition counseling unless the patient seeks mental health care. "We have come to a point where continuing to meet will not move things forward. I have to insist that you have at least one meeting with a counselor before we set our next appointment. After that meeting, have your counselor call me. Then we will get back together and keep pressing on."
- Manage your own feelings. Even if you insist, the patient may not see a counselor. You have made a referral and your patient must choose whether to pursue recovery. If you feel that you are abandoning your patient, speak with a support person about these completely normal feelings. Allow yourself to grieve that your patient is struggling. Expressing your feelings to a trusted colleague or adviser can help prevent this situation from adversely affecting your ability to make future referrals.

ADDITIONAL MEMBERS OF THE TREATMENT TEAM

Depending on a patient's symptoms and needs, a variety of additional supportive professionals may be added over the course of treatment, either for evaluation and consultation, or on an ongoing basis. Table 11.1 lists potential team members to whom you or other members of the treatment team may refer your patients. Generally, it is appropriate to consult with or inform other members of the treatment team before or after you refer a patient for additional care.

Table 11.1 Supplementary Treatment Team Members

Team Member (Role)	*Indications*
Psychiatrist or psychiatric nurse practitioner (Evaluation, diagnosis, medication management)	Any eating disorder or psychiatric diagnosis
Dentist (Dental care)	Chronic vomiting; bruxism (teeth grinding); pain reported in the mouth, gums or oral cavity; gum disease or tooth loss due to malnutrition
Family therapist (Provide support to patient in communicating/improving relationships with family members)	Family members argue during or about nutrition counseling; family dynamics contribute to or perpetuate eating disorder behavior; family members not coping well with stress
Physical therapist, exercise physiologist, or other movement therapist (Exercise prescription; injury rehabilitation; stress management, relaxation, release of physical tension)	Patient has been medically approved to exercise; patient is recovering from injury; patient unaware of appropriate intensity/duration/mode of physical activity
Art therapist (Emotional access and healing through creative expression)	Difficulty with self-expression in talk therapy
Religious leader (Spiritual healing)	Religious beliefs or conflict with God/higher power impairing recovery; history of religious abuse (religion used to promote guilt or shame in childhood)
Cardiologist (Cardiac care, medical clearance for physical activity)	Chest pain, palpitations, shortness of breath; rapid/significant weight loss; personal or family history of heart disease

(continues next page)

Table 11.1 Supplementary Treatment Team Members (continued)

Team Member (Role)	*Indications*
Endocrinologist (Hormone evaluation, insulin resistance, diabetes management)	Irregular menstrual cycle not attributed to malnutrition; failure to achieve menarche by 17 years of age; substantial weight gain at menarche or menopause; infertility; diagnosis or potential symptoms of diabetes, hypo- or hyperthyroidism, polycystic ovary syndrome, or other endocrine disorder
Gastroenterologist (Digestive care)	Chronic vomiting and/or laxative abuse; blood in stool or vomit; chronic/severe unexplained abdominal pain; reflux; diagnosis or symptoms of celiac disease, Crohn's disease, or irritable bowel disease; chronic/severe constipation
Speech therapist/pathologist (Feeding evaluation)	Difficulty chewing and/or swallowing food/beverages; repeated choking; aversion to eating after surgery or procedure
Group therapist (Support group leader)	Poor social support network; desire for peer interaction

DISCHARGE AND TRANSFER TO A NEW SETTING

Transitions in care occur for many reasons, such as when a patient leaves for college, moves to a new town, or simply wishes to change providers. However, the most common transitions for eating disorder patients are from a hospital or treatment center to a community-based setting or vice versa.

The decision to change the level of care is usually a joint decision of the members of the treatment team and the patient, together with family members, and possibly with input from the health insurance provider. The typical levels of care recognized in eating disorder treatment are listed in the following sections.

OUTPATIENT CARE

Outpatient care involves individual appointments with care providers in an office or clinic setting. Patients appropriate for this level of care meet the following criteria:

- Medically stable and in at least fair general health, requiring infrequent monitoring of weight and/or vital signs
- Self-motivated toward recovery and in a stable and supportive living environment
- Able to travel to and from scheduled appointments safely and reliably
- Able to follow a meal plan at home or at school (100% compliance not required)
- Able to resist purging, exercise, and self-harm triggers at home (100% compliance not required)
- Not actively suicidal

INTENSIVE OUTPATIENT PROGRAM

Intensive outpatient treatment involves group meetings supervised by care providers in 2- to 4-hour increments several times a week. Patients appropriate for this level of care meet the following criteria:

- Medically stable and in at least fair general health, but possibly requiring weight and/or vital signs to be monitored more than once per week
- Self-motivated toward recovery and in a stable and supportive living environment

- Able to travel to and from group and individual meetings safely and reliably
- Able to follow a meal plan at home or at school (100% compliance not required)
- Able to resist purging, exercise, and self-harm triggers at home (100% compliance not required)
- Not actively suicidal

DAY TREATMENT

Also called "full-day outpatient care" or "partial hospitalization," day treatment involves individual and group treatment for most waking hours, most days of the week, and includes one or more supervised meals each day. Day treatment programs may operate during typical work or school hours, such as 8 AM to 4 PM, Monday through Friday. "Partial hospitalization" typically refers to spending 7 days a week in a hospital treatment program, including all meals, but returning home to sleep. Patients appropriate for this level of care meet the following criteria:

- Medically stable to leave the hospital or facility, but requiring weight and/or vital signs to be monitored daily
- Having difficulty following a meal plan without supervision at mealtimes
- Having difficulty resisting purging or self-harm triggers without supervision
- Self-motivated enough in treatment to attempt to avoid detrimental behaviors when unsupervised at home in a stable living environment
- Able to travel to and from the facility safely and reliably
- Not actively suicidal

RESIDENTIAL TREATMENT/TREATMENT CENTER

Sometimes referred to as "rehab," residential treatment takes place at a free-standing treatment facility, which may or may not be affiliated with a hospital and may or may not be devoted exclusively to eating disorder care. Patients appropriate for this level of care meet the following criteria:

- Medically compromised and requiring daily or constant monitoring of weight and/or vital signs
- Unable to travel safely or reliably to treatment
- In an unstable and/or unsupportive living environment
- Unable to follow a meal plan without supervision and external motivation
- Unable to resist purging or self-harm triggers without supervision and external motivation; requires supervision using the bathroom
- Resistant and/or uncooperative in recovery, requiring constant structure and external motivation to remain safe

INPATIENT HOSPITALIZATION

Inpatient hospitalization involves full hospital care in either a medical, psychiatric, or eating disorders unit. Patients appropriate for this level of care meet the following criteria:

- Medically unstable and requiring daily or constant monitoring of weight, vital signs and/or laboratory test values. See Box 11.3 (2) for signs of medical instability. (Patients who are psychiatrically impaired or chemically dependent may also require inpatient hospitalization even if they are not medically unstable.)

- Malnourished and/or refusing oral intake, possibly requiring nutrition support, and weight less than 75% of expected body weight (adults)
- Malnourished and/or refusing food or acute weight loss, even if weight is within normal limits (children)
- Purging and/or self-harming unless constantly supervised; may be actively suicidal; may secretly exercise if left unsupervised; requires supervision using the bathroom
- Resistant and/or uncooperative in recovery, requiring constant structure and external motivation to remain safe; actively attempting to sabotage medical/nutrition care

Box 11.3 Signs of Medical Instability

- Heart rate less than 40 beats per minute (adult) or 50 beats per minute (child or adolescent)
- Blood pressure less than 90/60mmHg (adult) or 80/50mmHg (child or adolescent)
- A drop in blood pressure greater than 10 to 20mmHg when rising from sitting to standing position
- Plasma glucose level less than 60mg/dL
- Serum potassium less than 3mEq/L
- Body temperature less than 97°F
- Dehydrated, hypokalemic, or hypophosphatemic, and/or experiencing hepatic, renal, or cardiovascular complications requiring acute treatment

Source: Data are from reference 2.

"STEP-DOWN" CARE, TRANSITIONAL LIVING, "HALFWAY" HOUSE, OR GROUP HOME

Upon leaving inpatient or residential treatment, patients may participate in a less-structured living situation intended to prepare them to return to their own homes and outpatient care. This level of care is especially important when the patient's home living situation is not stable or the patient will be living alone for the first time.

If the inpatient or residential facility does not provide step-down care, options may be available in the patient's home town. At this level of care, supervision varies by facility. Facilities may provide a combination of group or individual therapy, 12-step meetings, a case worker or on-site supervisor, communal meals, curfews, and drug screenings—or none of these. Some facilities are simply a safe place to live and practice recovery.

A patient appropriate for this level of care meets the standards for outpatient care (described previously in this chapter), with the exception of the stable home living environment.

Ideally, patients do not switch instantly from inpatient to outpatient care. Instead, they step down to a lower level of care over time, practicing their independent living skills without being totally self-reliant. This type of transitional living is common for individuals recovering from drug or alcohol dependence, but atypical for those recovering from eating disorders. Depending on the community resources available, patients may seek residential treatment away from home and then must find local providers on an outpatient basis in their home town.

When transitional living opportunities specifically for individuals in eating disorder recovery are not available, the move from residential to outpatient care can be a very difficult time period. A common misconception that contributes to this difficult adjustment is that patients discharged from inpatient or residential care are considered "cured" and no longer practicing their eating disorder. However, duration of treatment can be limited by health insurance providers, and patients may leave care before achieving a stable level of recovery or the ability to maintain it. Additionally, home life entails a higher level of stressors of all kinds, which can render the skills obtained in the sterile environment of a treatment center far less effective.

Because patients can regress in their recovery in the first few weeks after discharge, it is in their best interest to have outpatient care appointments scheduled prior to discharge. This allows the inpatient and outpatient RDs to communicate necessary and helpful information.

MATCHING A PATIENT TO AN EATING DISORDER TREATMENT FACILITY

At times you may be asked to recommend a treatment facility for a particular patient. You cannot possibly know all of the options, nor which would be the best for your patient. Ultimately, the facility selection must be a joint decision of the patient, involved family members, and treatment facility staff. You may offer guidance to your patient if you are familiar with particular facilities. However, empowering your patient to research his or her options is ideal. The more empowered a patient feels in choosing a treatment facility, the more engaged he or she may be once there. Box 11.4 provides some questions you can suggest to a patient or family member who asks for your advice in choosing among treatment options (3). Choose the questions that are applicable to each patient's situation.

Box 11.4 Questions to Evaluate Eating Disorder Treatment Facilities

- Does the facility accept patients who are medically unstable?
- Can the facility provide medical care or medical nutritional rehabilitation when indicated by the patient's needs?
- What is the facility's philosophy of treatment, nutrition, and eating disorders?
- Does the facility help patients find follow-up care?
- What does treatment cost? What insurance coverage is available? Are payment plans available? Are charity beds available?
- What are the criteria for discharge? What is the average length of stay?
- Is the facility for patients with eating disorders only or for all types of psychiatric care?
- Does the facility provide treatment for additional issues that patients may have, such as trauma, substance abuse, or self-harm?
- Are visitors allowed? Do visitors or family members participate in treatment?
- Does the facility have a particular religious affiliation?
- Does the facility offer a step-down or transitional living program?

Source: Adapted with permission from Setnick J. *The Eating Disorders Clinical Pocket Guide: Quick Reference for Healthcare Providers.* Dallas, TX: Snack Time Press; 2005.

REIMBURSEMENT ISSUES

Obtaining insurance coverage for eating disorder treatment is rarely straightforward and can require many exchanges back and forth between insurance personnel, the insured, and members of the treatment team. The following are among the issues that make reimbursement challenging:

- An evidence-based treatment method for eating disorders has not been identified. Research is at times difficult to translate into clinical practice and vice versa (4–7). However, insurance providers hesitate to cover procedures and treatments without "proof" that they are effective (8).
- The view persists that eating disorder behaviors are a matter of choice or will, even though the biological basis has been confirmed (5).
- Benefits for mental health care coverage are not always adequate for the lengthy course of treatment that patients may require.
- Insurers waver on whether nutrition therapy for a mental illness is "medically necessary," even though American Psychiatric Association guidelines indicate that it is (2).

If you work in a facility, payment for your services may be rolled into a single per diem charge. You may never know whether your services are being directly reimbursed or paid for by insurance, and you may not need to know.

For RDs working in their own practices, reimbursement is more complicated. Even if you are a provider contracted with an insurance plan, reimbursement may still depend on each patient's diagnosis, covered benefits, and deductible amount.

RDs who are not contracted with an insurance company are out-of-network providers. When no in-network RD is available, ad-hoc coverage or a single-case agreement may be possible if the patient requests it from the insurance company. When a patient requests that a third party, such as an insurance company, pay for treatment, the RD and other team members may be asked to provide documentation for services rendered and their medical necessity.

The American Dietetic Association and other eating disorder advocacy organizations (see Appendix A) are working on many levels to obtain better insurance reimbursement for RD services and eating disorder treatment. Even when coverage is not guaranteed or expected, it is worthwhile to encourage patients to file their insurance claims, because such claims alert the insurance company that nutrition services are being used and increase awareness of the RD's essential role in eating disorder treatment.

REFERENCES

1. Kellogg M. When and how to refer to psychotherapy. *Weight Management Matters.* 2008;6(2):14–15.
2. Yager J, Devlin MJ, Halmi KA, Herzog DB, Mitchell JE, Powers P, Zerbe KJ. *Practice Guideline for the Treatment of Patients with Eating Disorders.* 3rd ed. Arlington, VA: American Psychiatric Association; 2006.
3. Setnick J. *The Eating Disorders Clinical Pocket Guide: Quick Reference for Healthcare Providers.* Dallas, TX: Snack Time Press; 2005.
4. Barnes S, Schwartz MB. Increasing collaboration between clinicians and researchers. *Renfrew Perspect.* 2007;(Winter):5–7.
5. Tobin DL. Research and practice in eating disorders: the clinician's dilemma. *Renfrew Perspect.* 2007;(Winter):8–10.
6. Kaye W, Grefe L. Why eating disorders research is underfunded. *Renfrew Perspect.* 2007;(Winter):3–5.
7. Banker J, Klump K. Toward a common ground: bridging the gap between research and practice in the field of eating disorders. *Renfrew Perspect.* 2007;(Winter):12–14.
8. Bunnell D. Evidence-based practice: an insurer's perspective. Interview with Andrei-Claudian Jaeger, MD, Medical Director, MHN, New York and New Jersey Service Center. *Renfrew Perspect.* 2007;(Winter):10–12.

Appendix A

Guide to Restrictive Eating Styles

RESTRICTIVE EATING STYLES AND EATING DISORDER TREATMENT

As with any patient population, patients with eating disorders may adhere to restricted eating styles for a variety of reasons. Rationale for these eating restrictions varies and may include desire for weight loss, religious tradition, medical necessity, family practices, disease prevention, personal moral and ethical beliefs, environmental concerns, and personal preferences.

In the context of eating disorders and eating disorder recovery, the line between appropriate and inappropriate dietary restrictions may be blurred—restrictions may consciously or subconsciously mask irrational beliefs about food and weight gain. It may take time for each patient, with your help, to pick apart the true rationale behind dietary restrictions and whether to continue them during recovery.

Depending on how and why a particular patient applies food restrictions, you may determine that the restrictions are not nutritionally adequate or appropriate to promote recovery. Each facility should have a standard policy in place for handling patient food preferences at admission so that patients and their involved family members can make informed decisions about whether their dietary needs can be met during treatment, or if they are willing to relax their dietary standards for the duration of stay at that facility.

The treatment team should always give respect to a patient's personal preferences. However, if it is in the patient's best interest to include some formerly excluded foods, this topic can be appropriately broached by the registered dietitian. Most eating styles, including those founded on religious beliefs, allow latitude in light of medical needs. Islam allows members of the Muslim faith to eat non-halal food if halal food is not available, and Judaism forbids fasting on fast days for Jewish patients whose health will be harmed by fasting. Patients who are struggling with religious beliefs that conflict with their eating disorder treatment may benefit from referral to a religious leader of their faith who can help reconcile the conflict or grant "permission" to follow medical advice that seems to contradict with religious teachings.

The following sections describe a variety of restrictive eating styles. In some cases, a patient may not accurately or strictly follow the restrictive eating style to which he or she subscribes. It is therefore important to investigate each patient's actual food preferences so that the meal plan is not unnecessarily restricted. In addition, patients may be willing to relax eating standards temporarily in the interest of recovery.

PLANT-BASED EATING STYLES

Rationales

A patient's rationale for following a plant-based eating style could be health-related, political (eg, animal rights–based), or linked to a past bad experience with a meat-based food. The following table lists types of vegetarian/ vegan eating styles.

Eating Style	*Excluded Animal Foods*	*Included Animal Foods*
Semi-vegetarian	Beef, pork, and products made from these meats	Poultry, eggs, seafood, and dairy
Pesco-vegetarian	Beef, pork, poultry, and products made from these meats	Seafood, possibly dairy, and eggs
Lacto-ovo vegetarian	Beef, pork, poultry, meat products, and seafood	Dairy and eggs
Lacto-vegetarian	Beef, pork, poultry, meat products, seafood, and eggs	Dairy
Vegan	All foods provided by animals including honey	Plant-based foods only

Macrobiotic Eating Style

The macrobiotic eating style is shaped by a philosophical desire to live "in balance with nature" for a healthy mind, body, and spirit.

- **Excluded foods**: all animal products, certain fruits and juice, coffee, processed foods, and artificial ingredients
- **Included foods**: beans, vegetables, tofu, whole grains, and tea.

Raw Foods Eating Style

This eating style is based on the belief that heating foods destroys their digestive enzymes and that cooking diminishes the nutritional value and "life force" of food.

- **Excluded foods**: cooked food, processed food, and food heated to 116°F or higher
- **Included foods**: raw vegetables, fruits (fresh or dried), sprouts, nuts, seeds, grains, beans, and seaweed

CALORIE-RESTRICTING EATING STYLE

The calorie-restricting eating style is an effort to prolong lifespan. Daily caloric intake is restricted to at least 10% below estimated energy needs.

- **Excluded foods**: processed sugars and flour; red meat; and white rice
- **Included foods**: vegetables and small amounts of fish. Nutrition supplements are also allowed.

KASHRUS EATING STYLE

The kashrus eating style is also called "keeping kosher" or "kosher." The food choices are governed by Jewish religious belief prescribed in the Old Testament. Kashrus is not followed by everyone of the Jewish faith, and individuals adhere to the rules to varying degrees. For example, some individuals will not eat any foods prepared in a non-kosher kitchen, but others are less strict about this. Assess choices and restrictions on an individual basis before ordering a kosher meal plan for a patient.

- **Excluded foods**: pork and all pork products (including products containing pork gelatin); shellfish; and

beef and poultry that are not certified kosher. Dairy and meat of any kind cannot be included in the same meal.
- **Included foods**: all fruits and vegetables, dairy products, and fish; beef and poultry certified kosher; and packaged food labeled with kosher symbols.

Depending on their level of religious observance, Jewish patients may or may not adhere to additional religious food restrictions throughout the year. On Passover, bread and many products made from grains are not eaten. On Yom Kippur, abstaining from all food and beverages is required by anyone 13 years or older. Ideally, these observances should be temporarily waived if they have previously been related to the eating disorder or if following them would impair the progress of recovery.

HALAL EATING STYLE

The halal eating style is based on Muslim religious beliefs prescribed in the Koran. Halal is not followed by everyone of the Muslim faith, and there are varying degrees of adherence. Assess food choices and restrictions on an individual basis.

- **Excluded foods**: pork and all pork products (including pork gelatin) and alcohol in any form
- **Included foods**: all fruits and vegetables, dairy products and fish, as well as beef and poultry certified halal or kosher

Depending on their level of religious observance, Muslim patients may or may not adhere to additional religious food restrictions throughout the year. During the month of Ramadan, fasting during daylight hours is observed. Ideally, these observances should be temporarily waived if they have previously been related to the eating disorder or if following them would impair the progress of recovery.

RESTRICTIVE EATING DURING LENT

Orthodox Christian Lent Eating Style

During Lent, Orthodox Christianity prohibits the consumption of animal foods during Lent (the time period from Ash Wednesday through Easter), except on Sundays when food choices are unrestricted. Level of religious observance varies; evaluate on an individual basis.

Catholic Lent Eating Style

Catholicism prohibits the consumption of meat from hooved animals (ie, beef and pork) on Fridays during Lent (the time period from Ash Wednesday through Easter). Fish and dairy are allowed on Fridays, and food choices on other days are unrestricted. Level of religious observance varies; evaluate on an individual basis.

Protestant Lent Eating Style

Individuals of certain Protestant faiths choose something to "give up for Lent," the period from Ash Wednesday through Easter. Many will give up a food, but this is not a requirement.

People can choose to stop an activity, such as gossiping or another bad habit. Level of religious observance varies; evaluate on an individual basis.

GLUTEN-FREE EATING STYLE

The gluten-free diet is a medical diet for celiac disease (gluten intolerance), which has been adopted by celebrities and become a fad diet touted for weight loss and general health. Following a gluten-free diet before diagnosis with celiac disease can confound test results and cause a false negative reading.

- **Excluded foods**: wheat, rye, barley (all of which contain gluten) and all foods containing them, their flour, or their gluten-storage proteins, gliadin, secalin, and hordein. This restriction excludes most baked goods, pastas, and cereals, as well as numerous processed foods with ingredients that contain gluten.
- **Included foods**: all meats, fish and seafood, poultry, eggs, corn, quinoa, rice, legumes, nuts, seeds, dairy, fruits, and vegetables, as well as baked goods, cereal, and pasta made from gluten-free flours; malt vinegar.

Appendix B

Caffeine Content in Common Foods, Beverages, and Drugs

Coffees

	Service Size, oz	*Caffeine/ Serving, mg*
Coffee, generic brewed (range: 102–200; 16 oz = 266)	8	133
Starbucks brewed coffee (grande)	16	320
Einstein Bros. regular coffee	16	300
Dunkin Donuts regular coffee	16	206
Starbucks vanilla latte (grande)	16	150
Coffee, generic instant (range: 27–173)	8	93
Coffee, generic decaffeinated (range: 3–12)	8	5
Starbucks espresso (doppio)	2	150
Starbucks Frappuccino blended coffee beverages, average	9.5	115
Starbucks espresso, solo	1	75
Einstein Bros. espresso	1	75
Espresso, generic (range: 30–90)	1	40
Starbucks espresso decaffeinated	1	4

Teas

	Service Size, oz	*Caffeine/ Serving, mg*
Tea, brewed (range: 40–120)	8	53
Starbucks Tazo Chai tea latte (grande)	16	100
Snapple, Lemon (and diet version)	16	42
Snapple, Peach (and diet version)	16	42
Snapple, Raspberry (and diet version)	16	42
Arizona Iced Tea, black	16	32
Nestea	12	26
Snapple, Just Plain Unsweetened	16	18
Arizona Iced Tea, green	16	15
Snapple, Kiwi Teawi	16	10

Soft Drinks[a]

	Service Size, oz	*Caffeine/Serving, mg*
Vault	12	71 (20 oz = 118 mg)
Jolt Cola	12	72
Mountain Dew MDX, regular or diet	12	71 (20 oz = 118 mg)
Coke Black	12	69 (20 oz = 115 mg)
Coke Red, regular or diet	12	54 (20 oz = 90 mg)
Mountain Dew, regular or diet	12	54 (20 oz = 90 mg)
Pepsi One	12	54 (20 oz = 90 mg)
Mellow Yellow	12	53
Diet Coke	12	47 (20 oz = 78 mg)

(continues next page)

Soft Drinks[a] (continued)

Diet Coke Lime	12	47 (20 oz = 78 mg)
TAB	12	46.5
Pibb Xtra, Diet Mr. Pibb, Pibb Zero	12	41 (20 oz = 68 mg)
Dr. Pepper	12	42 (20 oz = 68 mg)
Dr. Pepper diet	12	44 (20 oz = 68 mg)
Pepsi	12	38 (20 oz = 63 mg)
Pepsi Lime, regular or diet	12	38 (20 oz = 63 mg)
Pepsi Vanilla	12	37
Pepsi Twist	12	38 (20 oz = 63 mg)
Pepsi Wild Cherry, regular or diet	12	38 (20 oz = 63 mg)
Diet Pepsi	12	36 (20 oz = 60 mg)
Pepsi Twist, diet	12	36 (20 oz = 60 mg)
Coca-Cola Classic	12	35 (20 oz = 58 mg)
Coke Black Cherry Vanilla, regular or diet	12	35 (20 oz = 58 mg)
Coke C2	12	35 (20 oz = 58 mg)
Coke Cherry, regular or diet	12	35 (20 oz = 58 mg)
Coke Lime	12	35 (20 oz = 58 mg)
Coke Vanilla	12	35 (20 oz = 58 mg)
Coke Zero	12	35 (20 oz = 58 mg)
Barq's Diet Root Beer	12	0
Barq's Root Beer	12	22 (20 oz = 38 mg)
7-Up, regular or diet	12	0
Fanta, all flavors	12	0
Fresca, all flavors	12	0

(continues next page)

Soft Drinks[a] (continued)

Mug Root Beer, regular or diet	12	0
Sierra Mist, regular or free	12	0
Sprite, regular or diet	12	0

[a]The Food and Drug Administration (FDA) official caffeine limit for cola and pepper soft drinks is 71 mg per 12 oz.

Energy Drinks

	Service Size, oz	*Caffeine/ Serving, mg*
Spike Shooter	8.4	300
Cocaine	8.4	288
Monster Energy	16	160
Full Throttle	16	144
Rip It, all varieties	8	100
Enviga	12	100
Tab Energy	10.5	95
SoBe No Fear	8	83
Red Bull	8.3	80
Red Bull Sugar-free	8.3	80
Rockstar Energy Drink	8	80
SoBe Adrenaline Rush	8.3	79
Amp	8.4	74
Glaceau Vitamin Water Energy Citrus	20	50
SoBe Essential Energy, Berry or Orange	8	48

Frozen Desserts

	Service Size, fl oz	*Caffeine/ Serving, mg*
Ben & Jerry's Coffee Heath Bar Crunch	8	84
Ben & Jerry's Coffee Flavored Ice Cream	8	68
Haagen-Dazs Coffee Ice Cream	8	58
Haagen-Dazs Coffee Light Ice Cream	8	58
Haagen-Dazs Coffee Frozen Yogurt	8	58
Haagen-Dazs Coffee & Almond Crunch Bar	8	58
Starbucks Coffee Ice Cream	8	50-60

Chocolates, Candies, and Other Foods

	Service Size	*Caffeine/ Serving, mg*
Jolt Caffeinated Gum	1 stick	33
Hershey's Special Dark Chocolate Bar	1.45 oz	31
Hershey's Chocolate Bar	1.55 oz	9
Hershey's Kisses	41 g (9 pieces)	9
Hot Cocoa	8 oz	9 (range: 3-13)

Over-the-Counter Drugs

	Dosage	*Caffeine/ Serving, mg*
NoDoz (Maximum Strength)	1 tablet	200
Vivarin	1 tablet	200
Excedrin (Extra Strength)	2 tablets	130
Anacin (Maximum Strength)	2 tablets	64

Source: All tables in this appendix are adapted with permission from Caffeine Content of Food and Drugs. Center for Science in the Public Interest Web site. September 2007. http://www.cspinet.org/new/cafchart.htm. Accessed August 10, 2010. (Most information was obtained from company Web sites or direct inquiries. Serving sizes are based on commonly eaten portions, pharmaceutical instructions, or the amount of the leading-selling container size. For example, beverages sold in 16-oz or 20-oz bottles were counted as one serving. Additional information: Juliano LM, Griffiths RR. Caffeine. In: Lowinson JH, Ruiz P, Millman RB, Langrod JG, eds. *Substance Abuse: A Comprehensive Textbook*. 4th ed. Baltimore: Lippincott, Williams, & Wilkins; 2005:403–421.)

Appendix C

Additional Resources

BOOKS, WORKSHOPS, AND OTHER RESOURCES FOR AND BY REGISTERED DIETITIANS TREATING EATING DISORDERS

Brannon-Quan T, Licavoli L. *Love Your Body: Change the Way You Feel About the Body You Have.* Carlsbad, CA: Gurze Books; 2007. www.bulimia.com

Clark N. *Nancy Clark's Sports Nutrition Guidebook.* 4th ed. Champaign, IL: Human Kinetics; 2008. www.nancyclarkrd.com

Curry KR, Jaffe A. *Nutrition Counseling and Communication Skills.* Philadelphia, PA: WB Saunders; 1997.

Eberle SG. *Endurance Sports Nutrition.* 2nd ed. Champaign, IL: Human Kinetics; 2007. www.eatdrinkwin.com

Ekvall SW, Ekvall VK, eds. *Pediatric Disorders in Chronic Diseases and Developmental Disorders: Prevention, Assessment, and Treatment.* 2nd ed. New York, NY: Oxford University Press; 2005.

Herrin M. *Nutrition Counseling in the Treatment of Eating Disorders.* 2nd ed. New York, NY: Brunner-Routledge; 2003.

Johnston AJ. Tending the Feminine Psyche annual workshop. www.DrAnitaJohnston.com.

Kellogg M. Molly Kellogg's Counseling Intensive Workshop for Nutrition Therapists and *Counseling Tips for Nutrition Therapists Practice Workbooks* vol. 1 and 2. www.mollykellogg.com

Kostas GG. *The Cooper Clinic Solution to the Diet Revolution.* 2009. www.georgiakostas.com

Kratina K, King N, Hayes D. *Moving Away from Diets: Healing Eating Problems and Exercise Resistance.* 2nd ed. Lake Dallas, TX: Helm Publishing; 2003. www.helmpublishing.com

Kronberg S. *Comprehensive Learning Teaching Handouts.* Carlsbad, CA: Gurze Books. www.bulimia.com

Myers ES. *Winning the War Within: Nutrition Therapy for Clients with Eating Disorders*. 2nd ed. Lake Dallas, TX: Helm Publishing; 2008. www.helmpublishing.com

Pereya L. Forms, handouts and worksheets for work with eating disorders. Nutritious Ways Web site. www.nutritiousways.com

Pronsky ZM, Crowe JP. *Food-Medication Interactions*. 16th ed. Birchrunville, PA: Food-Medication Interactions; 2010. www.foodmedinteractions.com

Setnick J. *Eating Disorders Boot Camp Training Workshop for Professionals Home-Study Course*. www.understandingnutrition.com

Tribole E, Resch E. Intuitive Eating: *A Revolutionary Program That Works*. New York, NY: St. Martin's Press; 2003. (Authors also provide professional training. For information, go to Intuitive Eating Web site: www.intuitiveeating.com.)

EATING DISORDER ORGANIZATIONS

Academy of Eating Disorders: www.aedweb.org

Binge Eating Disorder Association: www.bedaonline.com

Eating Disorder Hope (resources for coping with eating disorders): www.eatingdisorderhope.com

EatingDisorderJobs.com (resources for professionals and jobseekers): www.eatingdisorderjobs.com

Eating Disorder Referral and Information Center: www.edreferral.com

Eating Disorders Coalition: www.eatingdisorderscoalition.org

Gurze Books Eating Disorders Catalog: www.bulimia.com

International Association of Eating Disorder Professionals: www.iaedp.com

MentorConnect (eating disorders mentoring community): www.mentorconnect-ed.org

National Association for Men with Eating Disorders: www.namedinc.org

National Eating Disorders Association: www.nationaleatingdisorders.org

The Renfrew Center Foundation: www.renfrew.org

Index

Page number followed by *b* signifies box; *t,* table.